EXERCISES FOR **TRUE NATURAL** CHILDBIRTH

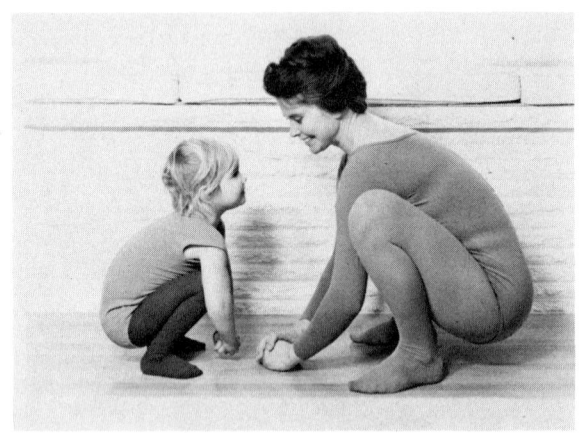

Photographs by Nicholas De Sciose and Gene Hinrichs

HARPER & ROW, PUBLISHERS

NEW YORK • EVANSTON • SAN FRANCISCO • LONDON

Rhondda Evans Hartman
B.S., R.N.

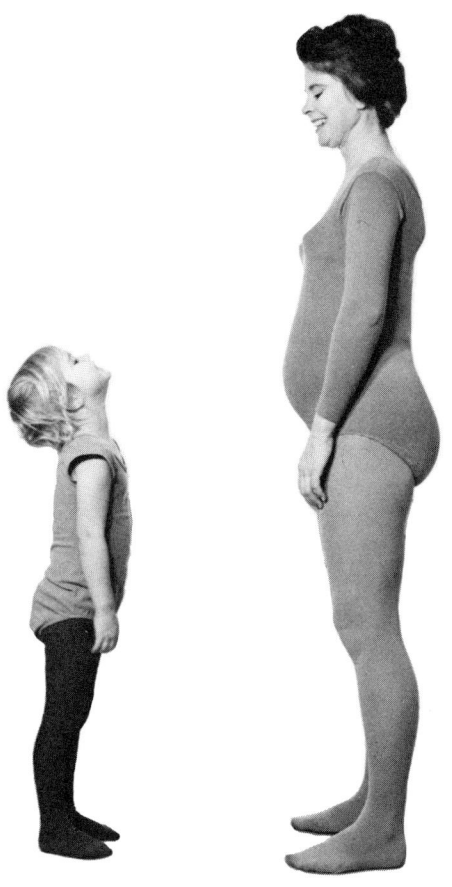

EXERCISES FOR **TRUE NATURAL** CHILDBIRTH

The cartoon on page 126, "Grin and Bear It" by George Lichty, courtesy of Publishers-Hall Syndicate.

EXERCISES FOR TRUE NATURAL CHILDBIRTH. Copyright © 1975 by Rhondda E. Hartman. All rights reserved. Printed in the United States of America. No part of this book may be used or reproduced in any manner whatsoever without written permission except in the case of brief quotations embodied in critical articles and reviews. For information address Harper & Row, Publishers, Inc., 10 East 53rd Street, New York, N.Y. 10022. Published simultaneously in Canada by Fitzhenry & Whiteside Limited, Toronto.

FIRST EDITION

Designed by Gwendolyn O. England

Library of Congress Cataloging in Publication Data

Hartman, Rhondda Evans.
   Exercises for true natural childbirth.

   1. Prenatal care. 2. Exercise. 3. Childbirth.
I. Title. [DNLM: 1. Gymnastics. 2. Natural childbirth. WQ150 H333e]
RG525.H27   1975   618.2'4   74–1814
ISBN 0–06–011766–4

---

75 76 77 78 79 10 9 8 7 6 5 4 3 2 1

*Dedicated to Dick
with love*

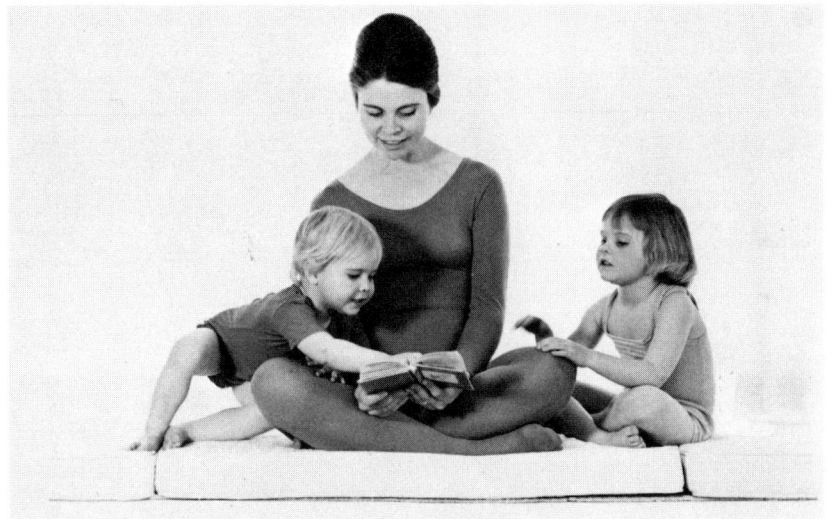

*Every child born into the world
Is a new thought
Of God,
An ever fresh and
Radiant possibility.*
　　　　　—KATE DOUGLAS WIGGIN

Contents

Foreword *by Dr. Robert A. Bradley*   ix

Preface by *Richard E. Hartman*   xiii

How to Use This Book   xv

Five Case Studies   1

Class One   15
- *Tailor Sit*   21
- *Pelvic Rock*   25
- *Relaxation*   29
- *Abdominal Breathing*   36
- *Squat*   40

Class Two   45
- *Leg Cramps*   46
- *Heartburn*   47
- *Eating for Two*   48
- *Variations of Pelvic Rock*   52
- *Sitting Pelvic Rock*   53
- *Standing Pelvic Rock*   55
- *Kitchen Sink Pelvic Rock*   58
- *Butterfly*   61

Class Three   64
- *Kegel Exercise*   65
- *Varicose Veins*   68
- *Leg Elevation*   70

Foot Circles 73
Leg Stretches 75
Breath Holding 77

Class Four 81
Breastfeeding 82
Bust Booster 88
Nipple Care 92

Class Five 95
How Labor Feels 96
Signs of Labor 97
False Labor 100
First-Stage Labor 101
Transition 104

Class Six 107
Second-Stage Labor 108
Birth 113
First Breastfeeding 114
Recovery Room 115
Hospital Stay 116
Going Home 117
Review 117

Postpartum 120
Being Parents 120
Being a Contented Mother 123
Tummy Tightener 127
Waist Trimmer 129
Being a Wife 130

A Letter to My Sister 133

Index 137

Foreword

Instinct is defined as "the innate propensity that incites animals to the actions that are essential for their existence, preservation, and development."

Human beings, though animals by virtue of our classification as mammals, apparently lack this innate propensity. As a result, we do not instinctively conduct our actions and behavior along pathways that will lead to preservation. Rather, from ignoring the great natural laws that manifest themselves automatically in the behavior of the other species of mammals in the bearing of their young to maintain and preserve their kind, we are not preserving but are gradually destroying our species, and even the environment and planet on which we live.

One pathway—and I consider it the most vital of all pathways to be preserved—is being destroyed as we bungle via drugs the reproduction of our species. Even before we clean up our external environment, we must first and foremost clean up the bloodstreams of our pregnant women, preventing their pollution with poisons and chemicals. Internal ecology must precede external, for drugs taken by pregnant women and laboring mothers have been proved to have deleterious effects on the brain and body functions of their offspring.*

Twenty-seven years ago, while in specialty training for obstetrics and gynecology, I proposed this as a theoretical possibility and earnestly suggested that human mothers, lacking instinct, should be trained to conduct themselves similarly to the other female mammals so that drugs and medications would be unnecessary in the reproduction of human babies. I felt not only that these drugs were temporarily harmful to newborn babies—which is obvious at just a cursory glance—but also that a subtle depletion of brain function persists throughout the lifetime of the individual.

I pointed out that by drugging mothers we are giving twenty times too large a dose to their unborn babies, as the baby receives the full dose of drug through the placental connection with the mother.

---

* See Robert A. Bradley, M.D., *Husband-Coached Childbirth*, rev. ed. (New York: Harper & Row, 1974).

Sir William Osler once stated that the main feature that distinguishes humans from other animals is the desire to take drugs.

Rhondda Hartman is a highly experienced teacher of true natural childbirth as well as being the mother of five husband-coached, unmedicated babies. She is a pioneer leader in the dawning of a new era of drugless childbirth, appropriately called "natural" childbirth, for what she teaches in this book is an exact copy of the instinctual behavior of similar mammals.

In following through my pet theory that you can teach humans how to perform "birthing" as well as, say, swimming—both actions being adroitly performed without instruction by all other mammals—I ran across innumerable obstacles, all of which can be overcome by the parents-to-be who carefully follow Mrs. Hartman's directions.

The first obstacle to overcome is that although people are designed amazingly like four-legged mammals, someone taught us to walk erect! As a consequence of this erect posture, not only do humans have unique problems, such as varicose veins on our "hind" legs, low backaches, toxemia of pregnancy, etc.—all of which are unheard of in our fellow mammals—but women's daily activities stiffen and weaken the muscles used in bearing babies.

The need for prenatal exercises to condition the childbearing muscles is thus obvious. I was delighted to have pointed out to me recently by an authority on whales and dolphins that these aquatic mammals go through a set pattern of daily prenatal exercises as soon as the female becomes pregnant, to strengthen their birth-giving muscles for later use.

Although it is fashionable now to assert that there is no difference between a man and a woman, I found this to be untrue in the demonstration of prenatal exercises. I needed women teachers to prepare women and Mrs. Hartman was one of the first to volunteer as a childbirth educator. She is not only a good teacher but is herself a shining example of what she teaches. In spite of her having borne five term babies, her body, as you can tell by the illustrations in this book, is beautiful, her posture perfect, and today she can join her grown children in ballet and modern dance performances. On a visit to Russia as a natural childbirth educator, she encountered skepticism that such a slim, lithe body had given birth to five babies. How does she maintain her good figure? She tells us in this book. To any pregnant woman I would say, "Do thou likewise."

Mrs. Hartman not only prepares the bodies of pregnant women, but because of her personal experiences so generously shared she further prepares the minds and souls of expectant mothers for the *joy* of childbirth. As vice-president of the American Academy of Husband-Coached Childbirth, she helps train and certify childbirth educators in the "Bradley Method" of true natural childbirth. The film of five births available from the academy is appropriately labeled "Childbirth for the Joy of It," for with proper preparation human "animals" can *enjoy* spontaneous, unmedicated births.

Young women today refuse to walk in the outmoded pathways of yesterday. They want their babies to be born without drugs, and they want to share the joyful experience of natural birth with their husbands. Woe be to any doctor who has the reputation of being a "drugger"— who administers medication routinely to unprepared patients. Woe be to any hospital so backward as to still be clinging to outmoded rules excluding husband-coaches.

The hope of a clean planet lies in the birthing without medication of intelligent, clear-brained babies who will grow up to solve our ecological problems. Not *more* babies but *better* babies result from following the example and teaching of this author, a true leader of a new and better generation. Let's get back to nature, obstetrically, before it is too late.

> Robert A. Bradley, A.B., M.D.
> President, American Academy
> of Husband-Coached Childbirth

Preface

"*It's a boy, it's a boy, a boy*, a boy, a boy!" I was shouting while jumping ten feet off the floor as our first-born, Joe, arrived—the culmination of nine months of eager anticipation.

I've been asked many times if the husband could possibly be as excited over natural childbirth as is his wife.

The word is: I still jump ten feet in the air at the memory of coaching my fantastically wonderful wife through five magnificent experiences resulting in five beautiful children.

Had it not been for Rhondda, I would have been gypped out of these powerful experiences, isolated in some lonely room out of communication, with suspicions that the worst was about to happen. As a matter of fact, I had given it little thought until Rhondda began educating me. Fortunately, Drs. Robert A. Bradley and Max D. Bartlett were pioneering in natural childbirth in my hometown, Denver. From the three of them I soon learned that a prospective father is important.

With the ultimate goal of a beautiful, healthy child in mind, I found that I could inspire my wife to train as an athlete and, with a little imagination, make her exercise and diet, and even help make her discomfort more tolerable. It made sense to me that since all great athletes—from Olympic skiers to competitive horseshoe players—need coaching to perfect their skill, and since developing and having a baby is essentially physical, a coach is indeed important. I found coaching especially valuable during the tiring long labor with our first child. Rhondda needed my constant chatter of: "Come on, Rhondda baby, relax"—"Float this one out"—"Gee, that's really great"—"I'm really proud of you"—"This has been going on for hours and you've been riding them out like a dream"—"You keep this up and you'll be writing a book"—"O.K., you're probably getting close to transition"—"This is going to be a little tough, but relax because you're about to push"—"You can ride it out—remember, this time it's a short one"—"Aren't you getting excited?"—"Hey, nurse, check this one's dilation—she's about to go to press!"

I have to confess that during those wee hours of the night I had a tendency to put my head down and fall asleep, under the impression that Rhondda really didn't need me. She corrected me later. My best efforts were most helpful and most needed as Rhondda reached transition—those last contractions before pushing begins. The most exciting time for both of us was the pushing. I found the participation in the miracle of birth and the anticipation of seeing my own child come into the world superlative and exhilarating. When the final moment of truth did come, I feel convinced I really did jump ten feet off the floor out of sheer pent-up excitement.

RICHARD E. HARTMAN

How to Use This Book

This book is an attempt to teach you, the reader, as I would if we could be in a class situation. I've tried to put our total class instruction on paper so that you will know how to prepare for your labor. My approach is strictly nonmedical and practical.

As I write, I feel as though I know you. So this is a very personal experience between us. Teaching has been the greatest joy of my working career, but writing it, instead of saying it, has turned out to be the hardest, longest "labor" I've ever had.

I suggest you read the text quickly and then use it very methodically, exercise by exercise, so that you will really have your body and muscles ready by full-term pregnancy. We have developed the sequence of preparation with you in mind. Some of the basic, important postures we want you to learn as soon as possible, which may be in your second or third month of pregnancy, so that you will have enough time to be really prepared by the time you have your baby. Other exercises or postures or "tricks" we offer you when you may be needing some relief from that pressure in the pelvis as the baby gets bigger and heavier. We leave the discussion of labor itself until you are quite close to delivery—six to eight weeks prior to due date. I have discovered in myself a strange detachment from serious acceptance of the labor until I am really faced with it. This seems a fairly common reaction. When it's time, we'll discuss labor, how it feels, and what to do. Before this, it is a theory which you gloss over. In those last few weeks, you begin to deal with it as fact. Even when you have had a prior birth experience that was beautiful, this is true; so accept it as I have in myself and others, and let us prepare you in general terms while we build your muscles. We'll get to the specific details of labor as you are ready to accept the very hard work that having a baby requires. It is not easy, but it is probably going to be the most wonderful work you will ever do.

This book has been written with hospital births in mind. I have many friends who are "into" home births and I am somewhat envious. There could be no more pleasant environment for a birth than in my own home, but I'm not a gambler, and I work with doctors who aren't, either. I cannot accept the risk involved in being away from emergency care if it is needed. If you plan a home birth, the training that I offer will be very helpful in your labor. Hospitals are making every effort to create a homelike atmosphere in the maternity wards. See what your hospital offers.

I read a great deal and expect many of you do. You will get new and valid ideas from any book you read. I have one requisite about reading for your "method" of childbirth. Pick one plan of attack and follow it! Read all you want during early pregnancy, then choose the method or theory which most appeals to you. Once you are committed to a method, follow through vigorously with preparation and into labor. What we offer is probably the most basic, most practical method there is. I believe that is the reason for its success. We do not give you any "busy work," only two easy, effective techniques.

I've made references to other books which I hope you'll read. The public library should carry these books, and if it doesn't, librarians will often buy a book for a library when it is requested by several people. I am not asking you to buy other books, and I've tried to give you sufficient information so that you can do nicely without other books. Some of you will want more specific information, which I have not attempted to give you. There are many, many good books on the detailed physiology of childbirth, and for that reason I have limited myself to the subjective preparation and sensations of having a baby. Rather than what *is* happening during childbirth, I've stressed how it feels. However, I've tried to answer "why" as well. My prayer is that I've answered your need. May you have a healthy and happy pregnancy and a joyful childbirth!

In these pages I refer only to the normal, uncomplicated pregnancy. That is my expertise. It is a fact that at least 90 percent of you can have your babies as I have described, requiring absolutely no analgesia or anesthesia prior to the birth of the baby. In our records, 3 percent of the total required Caesarean sections, 3.6 percent had unforeseen complications, and 93.4 percent achieved spontaneous, uncomplicated, unanesthetized births.* To provide a safe margin on our sample, we will round this off to 90 percent.

I have not dealt with complications because I know nothing about their management. That is what the doctor is trained to do. You can be

---

* Robert A. Bradley, M.D., *Husband-Coached Childbirth*, rev. ed. (New York: Harper & Row, 1974), p. 45.

a great help to your doctor by doing your part as well as you can—relax and work with your body. Even if a complication should occur, you will have done your best and helped the uterus to do its job. There are usually many hours in a labor, and only the last few minutes can be anesthetized if it becomes necessary, so all your training will be very helpful. Caesarean section patients may be allowed to go into labor. Ours almost always are, so they need to know how to relax.

In other words, natural childbirth training will be helpful to all —even if you happen to be one of that 10 percent who cannot achieve our ultimate goal. Your pregnancy will be more pleasant, too, with all this preparation.

I have purposely left out any mention of types of anesthesia, because it is my expectation that you will not need any. But have I led you to believe that having a baby is easy? No! My hope is that you will accept childbirth for what it is—labor! It is work going on in your body such as you've never experienced. I hope you will appreciate the forces and be in awe of what is happening during the birth process. If you are well prepared as a couple, you will not let those forces overwhelm you, but will work with them to accomplish the goal.

These nine months are a great period in your life. Enjoy and experience them to the fullest.

Classes will be taught differently by every teacher—even when we agree totally on goals, methods, and training. Teaching is an individual skill and will vary with the teacher's personality.

The arrangement of classes will differ, too, depending on what is best under the circumstances. The order that I've given to my class routine is only a suggestion for you to follow, if you are a childbirth educator. In our case, we work closely with the doctors, who hold four monthly lectures with films. The couples attend those together. The exercises are held once a month for six months. We have "women only" at the first four exercise classes and then husbands and wives together for Classes Five and Six. In addition, there are once-a-month checkups at the doctor's office until the eighth and ninth months of pregnancy, when the visits are once a week. We keep very close contact with our couples!

Classes are necessarily set up to fit the doctors' requirements, so the routine will be different for each doctor. Or you may attend independently organized classes, which train couples for many doctors. This, too, will impose a slightly different routine. The classes must fill the needs of their members. The ideals are absolute, but the form may vary.

Each class has a personality of its own. And, within each group, it's very interesting to see the change from one session to the next as you develop a feeling of unity among the class members. Teaching never becomes dull because every class is so different—and always fun!

If you are planning to begin teaching childbirth classes, this book, along with Dr. Bradley's *Husband-Coached Childbirth*, will give you good basic material. If you are interested in teacher training, we offer a course to qualify you through the American Academy of Husband-Coached Childbirth, P.O. Box 5224, Sherman Oaks, California 91413. The teacher training has been set up with our principles as a basis.

Dr. Bradley talks to fathers about childbirth in his book; I have concentrated on reaching mothers—but it is my hope that you will enjoy my book as a couple. Happy birth day!

Five Case Studies

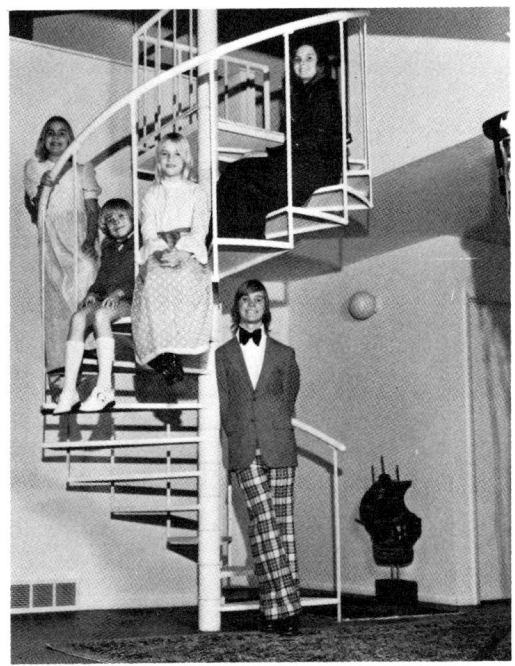

Joseph Baden
Claryss Nan
Rienne Frances
Allison Lucille
Richard Evans

Natural childbirth was about the furthest thing from my mind in 1956, when I was a young, single, just graduated public health nurse with a Bachelor of Science in Nursing from the University of Alberta, Canada. As a matter of fact, it was not a popular thought in very many minds. But five blooming young pregnant women came to me for help concerning natural childbirth as I started my public health career in the town of Lacombe, Alberta (population about 3,000). Their conviction inspired me to help them. My first approach was to go to their obstetrician for help but though he was very pleasant, he sent me on my way with a condescending "You're young yet, dear." My supervisor, Miss Edwina Buchan, to whom I went with all my problems, armed me with her blessings, a birth atlas, Maternity Center Association Guides for Teaching, and a phonograph record by Grantly Dick-Read, recorded while his patients were in labor. To those five young women I owe my interest in childbirth training. We all learned a great deal together but we lacked a very important ingredient—successful experience. We all benefited nonetheless.

That was my introduction to natural childbirth. Little did I know how it was to affect my life. My next assignment took me to Montreal, where I worked in a hospital and had no associations with pregnant patients, so the subject of natural childbirth was not important to me again until I became pregnant myself.

Since nothing is more personal than childbirth experiences, and that is my subject, I think it only right to tell you something of how I met my husband.

My friend Mary Mulloy (now Mrs. James Hawk) and I had saved and scrimped for a year and a half after graduation to buy steamship tickets to Europe. We went first to Portugal and Spain and spent a month touring before getting on another ship to cross the Mediterranean. It was on that ship I met Richard, a handsome, sophisticated lawyer from Denver, Colorado. It was love at first sight. After a chaotic, exciting, and romantic twelve days, our minds were made up (he took only five days, but I was more conservative), and six weeks after we had met we were married in Switzerland. The next five months we spent honeymooning in Europe and Canada in a tiny Fiat car that we bought in Zurich. It was glorious. What's more, we've never regretted our hasty decision!

Joseph Baden

In the natural course of events I found my interest in natural childbirth was revived. Richard and I began to seek an obstetrician soon after we settled in Denver, where his home and law practice were.

Richard, who had not given the birth process any thought, was puzzled when I announced we were going to have our child by natural childbirth. Even in a large major city, finding an obstetrician in 1958 who would know what "natural childbirth" meant required the services of a detective. (Some places have not changed!) Richard called his doctor friends, who scolded him for having such a foolish thought. Later, one of his doctor friends' nurses surreptitiously told him that to her knowledge there were only two doctors in the community who were sympathetic to the idea, Dr. Robert Bradley and his partner, Dr. Max Bartlett. Sympathetic was the understatement of the century. They were wildly excited and enthusiastic! Our first appointment completely sold Richard, who, as an attorney, cross-examined Dr. Bradley for about an hour. The pregnancy began to take on new dimensions as every question was answered in a complete, intelligent, and sensible manner. We were not hurried and he gave us all the time we needed to ask questions. At the interview, we learned that these doctors:

1. Took as patients only couples who wanted natural childbirth.
2. Gave medication only with complications or if absolutely necessary. They never asked if you "wanted" it, as it was a medical judgment (6 percent were given anesthetic, we were told).
3. Had their office next door to the Porter Memorial General Hospital, so they could run across the street to "catch" a baby at any given time.
4. Gave five lectures and films to each couple in large groups.
5. Had six exercise classes taught by their own trained obstetrical physiotherapist.
6. Expected husbands to share the total birth experience with their wives (including the delivery room) and would train them to coach their wives.

This was pure ecstasy. Suddenly, I had the full cooperation of the doctors and my husband as well. Richard became a salesman extraordinaire, convincing friends and neighbors, legal associates, and even strangers that they should use this sensible approach to having babies. The mystery, taboos, and magical aura were stripped away from the beautiful, functional thing that birth is meant to be.

We began going to the lectures and classes. Learning and doing. There were a few rough moments. One day I went to the office for my sixth-month checkup and Dr. Bradley, who has been known to be abrupt, discovered I was wearing a girdle. Well! The office fairly heaved and rumbled as he ranted and raved at me. Had I been attending classes? Why would I wear a blankety-blank thing like that? Did I want to be tied and hoisted into whalebone and rubber as my grandmother had been? What possible good was this doing for the baby? Did I need rubber to replace my own muscles? And so on and on! I stumbled out of his office defiantly wearing my girdle, with tears welling up in my eyes. After spilling my tears to my dear sounding-board husband, I realized that of course Dr. Bradley was right. I've never worn a girdle since that time, and after five children and a minimum of exercise, I have no bulge and a very flat stomach (my husband's editorial comment). There is no question about it: you do develop better muscle control when there is nothing holding you in but your own muscles.

Next, I had to learn some new habits, such as not crossing my legs when sitting; sitting on the floor tailor fashion whenever possible instead of in a chair; never getting into bed without doing pelvic rocks; resting with my feet up while lying down for some part of the day; and in general getting my body in A-1 condition. This takes discipline. A loving, trained husband can help by insisting upon right habits. Richard always nagged me not to bend my back but to squat. He learned along with me to count protein grams to make sure our diet was adequate for growing a baby. He learned what abdominal breathing is and how to help me relax. He became very good at holding his breath for forty seconds along with me. It became *our* pregnancy—an event which we shared and learned about and prepared for together!

The lectures and films that the doctors presented answered most of our questions as pregnancy progressed, so the visits to the office were quick and to the point. The exercise classes taught by Peggy Rice were fun. We were able to laugh and talk as a group and discovered together how normal we all were. Here we learned exercises to prepare muscles for the work ahead and posture tips for the lightening of our load over nine months. It helped to see that others were doing natural childbirth since none of our friends even approved. We found that we *liked* the natural childbirth people!

You know, the most amazing part about my own pregnancy, even with my training and background as a registered nurse, is how little I knew about pregnancy. I greatly appreciated the fact that these doctors explained things to me without regard to my R.N. It's wonderful not to have to admit you don't know! This pregnancy was uncomplicated and happy. We were so glad to be sharing this adventure, which cannot help but bring a couple closer together.

On April 1, the day before my due date, my body was surging with energy. I should have remembered about the "nesting" instinct, which is a term we've borrowed from animal behavior. When they sense the onset of labor, they instinctively begin to prepare a nest for their young. A cat will frequently find a clothes hamper and move the contents to a quiet, dark closet, working until she has a comfortable nest in which to give birth to her kittens. Nature seems to provide extra energy for all this activity. We human beings are apt to misuse the energy which nature provides at the beginning of our labor. In my case it happened to coincide with the day we moved from my husband's bachelor apartment downtown, which did not allow children, to a little three-bedroom house in the suburbs. He and I moved our entire personal belongings, and though there was not all that much, looking back on it, it took strenuous work to transport ourselves from apartment to home. I expended Herculean energy without difficulty, but was glad to crawl into bed about midnight. Soon thereafter, I had a few contractions, but after carrying several tons of books what else could you expect? A little false labor, I thought. At 4 A.M. I was awakened with regular five-minute contractions. I walked around the house for about an hour to make sure they were real. Then about 5 A.M. we headed for the hospital. In true new-father fashion, Richard, who had lived in Denver for ten years, lost his way to the hospital and approached panic in his search to get me safely to the doctor. He needn't have worried. The contractions continued at five minutes apart and I was barely dilated, with plenty of time for the usual procedure of hospital admittance—Johnny shirt, enema, shave, questions, and so on.

I began my long vigil of relaxing with each contraction. Hurray! Hurray! It worked! Joy upon joy! All my fears and doubts about my own ability were quickly dispelled. All those people who said, "Just wait, dearie," could now be refuted. I was doing it and it worked as the doctors said it would work. On and on I relaxed for twelve hours after coming to the hospital. Too bad that I had not recognized my "nesting instinct" and had saved that surge of energy for birth rather than moving, but it had not occurred to me at the time. The new daddy was the one who became weary, and I found him fast asleep from time to time and a bit concerned for the long delay, which of course was not much of a delay at all. He had been hearing too many tales about childbirth from his friends, too. I do wonder how anyone can tolerate a labor without the calm, cool, and unhurried composure that relaxing and abdominal breathing give you. I was completely aware of the contractions, but was riding with them rather than fighting against them, and this was well worth the effort of the training. I found a long labor is easier in that you can get very good at what you are doing. The only disadvantage was my not being well rested before the onset of labor. I found that I could fall asleep between contractions, and then be roused by the next one enough to concentrate on relaxing, then back to snoozing again. I did become somewhat edgy as transition into second stage arrived, and here Richard took over my relaxation. His calm, soothing voice would remind me to relax and breathe abdominally. Without him during transition, natural childbirth might have gone down the drain.

In an instant, the whole thing changed around. I couldn't and didn't want to relax anymore. After my examination by the OB nurse, who said, "Just one more relaxing contraction," my doctor arrived. He said, "Go ahead and push." Now we were into the exciting part of having a baby. My tiredness was gone; I felt peppy and happy and was ready to work all night. How gratifying it was to *do* something after all these hours of doing "nothing." The months' practice in holding my breath for forty seconds was now proving to be worth the effort. It was amazing to feel the tremendous tension begin to gather in the uterine area of my abdomen as I inhaled and expelled my first two breaths. Then I gathered my third big breath, held it, pulled my knees up to my shoulders like levers, put my chin forward on my chest, and pushed with all my might—then I felt nothing. No tension. No pain. Nothing except good, hard work and exhilaration. This is one time you cannot be ladylike and a weak clinging vine. It is now that you remember your pioneer forebears and know that you are capable of intense physical effort. I put all my strength into each push and feelings of discomfort were nil. After several pushes in the labor room with my bed adjusted some to make the pushing easier (head of the bed and knees up higher), the doctor announced that our baby's head was beginning to show. When I pushed, I looked in the mirror and saw a little dark spot and, I thought, black hair. I was soon to learn that the hair was blond and almost nonexistent and it was its wetness that made it appear black. It was time to move from the labor room to the delivery room so the doctor could better attend to the birth. By now I was feeling far too excited and spunky to be wheeled in on my bed and I advised the doctor I would walk. He winked at a horrified nurse and we paraded out of the labor room and into the room they call delivery.

I might tell you that the delivery table, once you are on it with your legs in the supports, has the bottom dropped and the top slanted so your head and thighs will be nearly at a forty-five-degree angle. With each contraction I inhaled two huge breaths and exhaled them forcefully, then, taking the third breath, I would bring my knees toward my shoulders, put my chin on my chest, and push with steady hard pressure. Between pushes, I would catch my breath while relaxing and waiting for the next contraction, much as a runner would act after running one lap of a foot race. Richard, in the meantime, wearing cap and mask and gown, was sitting on a stool near the head of the table, ordinarily occupied by the anesthetist. His big role was to be the cheering section, as he mopped my brow with a sloshy wet cloth, which by the way feels glorious, and helped push my shoulders and head toward my chest to aid me in bearing down. I was very strong, our baby was very eager to be born, the coach was marvelous, and in a very short time I felt a sudden release. A flood of pleasure and sheer happiness swept through me: we had successfully completed the first nine months of our child's existence. My emotions led me to false conclusions, however, for I heard the doctor calmly say, "Now we have the head and with the next contraction we'll have the whole baby." Waiting for the next push seemed to be an eternity, but it was a very short time, possibly two minutes. The last contraction took almost no effort, since the head is the largest part of the baby. The shoulders, then the rest of him easily arrived. What a miracle! What excitement! Proud papa realized he had a son and he shouted it for all to hear. "A boy, a boy, a boy!" We had known it all along, as the baby already had a name, one from each grandfather, Joseph Baden.

This was a time for great happiness. There is nothing like it! Richard and I were talking excitedly while the doctor held our baby below the level of my body for a few moments until the cord stopped pulsating, which indicated to him that all the placental blood was in the baby's body, where it belonged. Then the doctor wiped and suctioned the loose mucus from his nose and mouth before he was placed on my now flat tummy. What a thrill to hold my own baby for the first time! We were laughing and crying together, proud and happy and thoroughly delighted with each other. At this opportune moment, the doctor had injected some Novocaine for the episiotomy repair. He had cut me during one of my pushes and I had not even known! It is startling how the pushing created a numbness so that no anesthetic had been necessary. Now the pushing was all over, and a local anesthetic was kindly given so the suturing of the perineum could be done without discomfort. By the time all this embroidering was done, the placenta was loosened and expelled. I would not have been aware of it at all had not the doctor, knowing we'd be interested, explained to us what was going on.

After changing to a fresh nightie, I was on my feet, proudly holding our new son in one arm, my other arm around my husband, both of us beaming with huge smiles. The doctor had now switched to his role as photographer, using our camera. I felt fantastically good. Walking was a relief after the strenuous work during the pushing. In addition, I still had a vast amount of excited energy. The memory of all this, the pride of my husband as he took my arm for the walk down the hospital corridor, are among my most precious possessions.

Next stop, the recovery room. What a beautiful place to run up a huge telephone bill calling everybody from coast to coast—California and Connecticut—and from top to bottom—Canada and Texas. Everyone had to know. New parents are generally insufferable, and we were perhaps the worst of the lot! For a couple of hours, the nurses frequently checked my blood pressure, pulse, and uterus—to make certain it was contracted and hard. All things were normal. The baby was brought in during this time for us to admire and hold. In 1959 a three-day hospital stay was routine and since this was my first experience, I did go to the maternity ward and was tucked into bed for the night. By this time it was 9 P.M. and I had done two days' work on a limited night's sleep. I was ready for a good rest. However, I awakened very early in the morning, before dawn, to listen to the birds and to contemplate my new role as a mother. What a timeless feeling it was to be carrying on the ancestral line and to be but a small fragment of eternity, and at the same time, the frightening weight on my heart of the responsibility I now held as the mother of a new life, a new individual unlike any ever known—unique and entirely different!

Joey and I spent two more days in the hospital. Everything went smoothly and the staff was very nice to me, but I was eager to get home and share our baby with Richard. We left for home with our precious bundle on the morning of my birthday. Of course, we stopped for a birthday lunch, cake and all, and the baby slept peacefully. I sat comfortably for more than an hour and wondered why there is so much fuss made about heat lamps and "stitches." This natural childbirth was paying dividends at every stage.

We were not very different from most new parents arriving home to the newly painted nursery. We held our baby between us, admired him, and asked each other, "What do we do now?" That did not last long as we launched into our new routine. I was breastfeeding, so that part was easily taken care of—though it took time. In fact, I spent all my time with my baby. The house and meals were secondary. Poor Richard came home many days in that first month to find little done; lots of baby care but not much homemaking. I gradually learned to manage everything but will never forget that period, and I do try to warn new mothers of it.

When Joey was six weeks old, I began training to teach for Dr. Bradley and Dr. Bartlett. I was truly gratified to have been invited to join them. Mabel Lumm Fitzhugh came to Denver at Dr. Bradley's invitation and she and Peggy Rice instructed me in the intricacies of teaching exercises. I began teaching in May 1959 and am still at it.

Claryss Nan

Being parents agreed with us and we could hardly wait to have another baby. Two years later, on March 1, 1961, Claryss Nan arrived. My labor began at a La Leche meeting at Mary Ann and Tom Kerwin's house. We called Richard to come and take me to the hospital. We were excited but also very relaxed and in control. I was comfortable moving about much longer into the labor than I had been with our first. Second-stage labor was different in that I was far more aware of the pressure of the baby against the perineum. Pushing was much faster this time and in no time we had delivered a beautiful "round-headed" girl. (Joey's head had been somewhat pointed, molded from the long labor.)

We were thrilled to have a girl. This time we had decided to do what the Kerwins had pioneered—come home right away with the baby. Mary Ann had had home deliveries in Chicago but since that was not allowed here, the doctors had agreed to a happy compromise. A nursing baby and mother could be released from the hospital two hours after birth if there were no complications.

After two hours in the recovery room, during which time our pediatrician, Dr. Mijer, checked the baby, we proudly took Claryss Nan home to Joey, who was just waking up. (He'd been asleep when I'd called Richard, so a sitter had been hired for the night.) Grandmother Hartman had come out by taxi and the baby-sitter, Stephanie Bergren, was getting ready for school. Joey thought he'd never seen anything so marvelous as that baby. We all agreed. The best part of going home with the new baby was the reaction of her two-year-old brother.

I felt terrific after this birth. Comparing it to the first time, I now realized that I had been tired and a little shaky when I brought Joey home. I could not restrain myself: I invited people in for coffee and baby viewing and showed off in various ways. My poor neighbors were a bit dumfounded.

Second babies are such a joy. Claryss Nan was so good and my experience in mothering helped. We enjoyed our two children so much that it was inevitable that Rienne Frances would come along. She did on January 15, 1963.

Rienne Frances

Rienne decided to announce her incipient arrival while I was conducting a La Leche meeting at my home. (My babies picked great company!) It was the only time my membranes ruptured in early labor. I'd had a few scattered contractions during the day but nothing definite. The meeting was over and we were visiting when suddenly I seemed to have no control and thought I was wetting my pants! I pulled my Kegel muscle as tightly as I could and it got me to the bathroom, where I realized what was happening. The last of the ladies left while Richard and I called Stephanie to come and baby-sit for the night. Claryss Nan must have sensed what was going on, for she woke up during our preparations and came into our bedroom as I was relaxing on the bed with a rather hard contraction. It disturbed her to see me take no notice of her so she pulled my eyelid open with her fingers. All that practice in relaxing was very important.

We were excited but did not break speed limits driving to the hospital. As I was being admitted in the hospital room, I realized that I was ready to push. I sent a ward clerk for Dick before he drove off into the night (it was midnight now) looking for a place to buy film. My messenger caught him in time and he was on hand, an able coach, as one-half hour after we arrived at the hospital door, Rienne Frances was born. She was pink and beautiful and just what her father had expected, whereas I had been sure it was a boy all those nine months. Mothers do not always know!

Our first pictures of Rienne were at two hours instead of two minutes, but thank heavens Dick was with me during delivery.

Again we enjoyed our baby at home by morning as Joey and Claryss Nan woke up. Again the baby-sitter was able to get off to school, the new baby being settled safely at home.

And again Mary Ann Kerwin delivered a huge, elegant gourmet dinner complete with birthday cake (we had enjoyed the same treat from the Kerwins for Claryss Nan's birth celebration). This is the very best birth gift you could ever give to the parents of a new baby.

I have taken an informal survey on third babies. By and large they are the easiest to bring into the world and the hardest to fit into the family. This has nothing to do with the child, only the mothers! Usually the oldest is now about four years old, still requiring help with many of the daily routines. Add to the four-year-old a two-year-old toddler who is at the most delightful stage of all (I think so anyway) but undeniably a handful, and now a brand-new baby who requires you twenty-four hours a day. You find that mothering is hard work. You now have more children than you have hands and voice commands must be obeyed. Consider the simple act of crossing the street and you see what I mean!

However, four-year-olds are becoming very "why" oriented, so a whole new world of conversing with our oldest child, Joe, was opening up. Each stage in a child's development seems more fun than the last (of course, there are also stages you can hardly wait for them to outgrow).

My theory on "stages" is that it depends upon the parents. I believe that if a parent is not threatened by a stage of development, there is no problem. If the mother or father is upset at not being obeyed, then twos are terrible. A two-year-old is testing and exploring everything—even your instructions and commands. *I* love the "terrible twos"! They aren't terrible at all, but challenging and exciting.

We had become a little cramped in our house by now and talked of finding a larger one. To hear Richard tell the story, it was all my idea. He says, "We were at a party one evening and I heard my wife announce that we'd be moving soon." Anyway, Rienne's first year included lots of house hunting and she grew to hate riding in a car, which our other two loved. It was one of my many "standards" about children that I had to change. By the time you've a family of three, every rule, pronouncement, generality, and prejudice that you've collected about children and parenting has been broken. We knew so much about raising children before we had any!

As Rienne was nearing her first birthday, we moved into a house with four bedrooms, one for us and one for each child. You know what happened. Our 97-percent-sure birth control put us in the other 3 percent!

Allison Lucille

Amazingly enough, my fourth pregnancy was easier than the third had been. I did not have so much pressure and thankfully I did not have so much heartburn. We were tied down to a routine now, with Joe in kindergarten and the car pool that went with it. I was very involved in baby business, teaching childbirth classes and leading La Leche League meetings. The nine months went by very quickly.

One early afternoon in April, I began to feel contractions which were regular but not too strong. I expected false labor by my fourth pregnancy and did not get too excited. It seemed a good idea to alert Dick that he might need to come home. So I called the office and told him that I was having light contractions and although they were less than ten minutes apart, I did not think it was time to go to the hospital. I'd call him when I wanted him home. He came home immediately.

By about 5 P.M. I gave in and we went to the hospital, to have the doctor tell us that although I was dilating, I could go home if we wanted until the labor picked up. We didn't want. Instead we took a "leave" from the hospital to go out for dinner. We went to a drive-in and I tried to avoid fried, greasy food. That's not easy. What I wanted was a soft-boiled egg and toast but I made do with a milk shake and hamburger. We took a drive over what seemed to be the bumpiest roads ever (every road is bumpy when you are in labor). I was ready to do anything to avoid going home to the family without a baby! We returned to the hospital and walked the halls awhile until finally my contractions increased in intensity. They had been rather close together all along—about four to five minutes apart. From about midnight until 5 A.M. I was in good, effective labor. The rest of the labor could probably be considered "false," but that's an objective decision. It seemed true when I was in it!

Allison Lucille was born at 5:08 A.M., April 27, 1965. She picked a great time of day to arrive because Dr. Mijer made his hospital rounds by 7 A.M. He checked her and we were able to go home in our customary two hours.

Our friends the Dannebergs tell this story about that morning. They phoned our house to find out how things were going and when I answered the phone they assumed that I'd been in false labor and had come home empty-handed. As Florence was sympathizing with my having had to go through all that false labor, I interrupted her to tell her we had a baby. There was dead silence on the telephone. To this day she can't get over my coming home with a two-hour-old baby! She sent over a beautiful dinner of fried chicken, though. Mary Ann Kerwin brought her traditional dinner, too, another day. We ate well with new little Allison!

Although I felt great, my need to show off had subsided. I enjoyed being at home with my new baby and my little family. I hated even to answer the phone. There is something so special about those first few days with a new baby. In a very short time, however, my idyll was over and it was back to car pooling, for kindergarten, and to shopping for groceries.

Allison taught me some new lessons in baby care. For one thing, a nice plump baby (eight pounds two ounces at birth) may want to change her growth patterns. The doctor ran all sorts of tests to check her health when she refused to gain weight. We both finally concluded that she was O.K. and we'd let her be the boss. She was one year old when she finally doubled her birth weight. (Most babies double by four to six months.) Bless Dr. Mijer for not being upset. Thank goodness she was our fourth and I'd already proved myself an able breastfeeding mother. Allison is still very slight though rather tall. She resists food unless it's her idea. It will help you as parents if you can accept that a baby comes to you with many individual personality traits already built in. Do not expect to "create" your child's personality. Just help it to flower and grow in the most positive way you can. I try to remember what our child psychologist friend Katherine Tennes says: "Parents take either too much credit or too much blame for their children."

Richard Evans

With our fourth pregnancy most of our friends tried to be politely pleased, but with the fifth there was general disapproval. My parents felt that I had enough to do and Dad had been telling us for two pregnancies to name the baby Sufficient. Nevertheless, we all looked forward to another baby. It becomes an addiction!

Since our due date for this baby was January 5, my parents decided to come for Christmas, from their home in Parkland, Alberta, and stay till the birth. We were delighted to finally share this experience with these grandparents. Grandmother Hartman had celebrated new babies with us three times.

My father still complains that Ritchie tricked us by delaying his birth ten days. Dad was anxious to get home!

This time I experienced false labor for sure. It is typical of "grand multips," as the mothers of several children are called. (Some, however, have babies more easily each time.) For three days and nights I had contractions twenty minutes apart. It was not uncomfortable but so discouraging! Dick and I went to a movie to pass the time; we went to a church annual meeting (where all the older ladies wanted to get me to the hospital immediately). Of course, I went to the doctor. His advice was go to bed and rest. Finally the contractions picked up to a ten-minute interval. We checked into the hospital at 10 P.M., fairly sure that the contractions would keep going this time. By about 3 A.M. I must have been in transition stage of labor, because though both Dick and the doctor were sleeping, I demanded their presence. The nurse didn't question my motives and called them. They dutifully sat with me for more than an hour of labor. Dick had rather a bad cold and had been doing a good coaching job for three days—so until my "witchy" transition personality, I had been perfectly content to let him rest.

At last my labor moved into the pushing stage and shortly thereafter our second son was born. Again my guess had been wrong and Richard's right. It was delightful to have another boy to even up our family a bit but it made the bedroom arrangement very complicated. (We have since remodeled.)

Richard Evans Hartman checked in on January 15, 1967, and when we took him home a few hours later, there was quite a welcoming committee. Two-year-old Allison was beside herself with ecstasy. Rienne was celebrating her fourth birthday and what little girl ever had a better birthday present? The grandparents were thrilled and incredulous at both their new grandchild and their own daughter, who could enjoy the birth of her baby and be home showing him off in two hours. Joe and Claryss Nan were old hands at this experience by now, but loved it all.

This child rides with the waves created by everyone else in the family. He has to! He can sit in the middle of the biggest hubbub and quietly play his own game.

There is something special about the last baby, as you try to appreciate everything to the fullest. As with my first, I have had two years "alone" with the last. As Allison went off to school, Ritchie and I had time together. So the attention he missed as the number five child has been made up for now. The children give each other a great deal of attention, too, although some of that attention is not of a very positive variety!

It's an exciting household we have and I feel fortunate to have our large family. We are also fortunate to have "discovered" natural childbirth and to have celebrated each birth. We are indeed blessed.

CLASS ONE

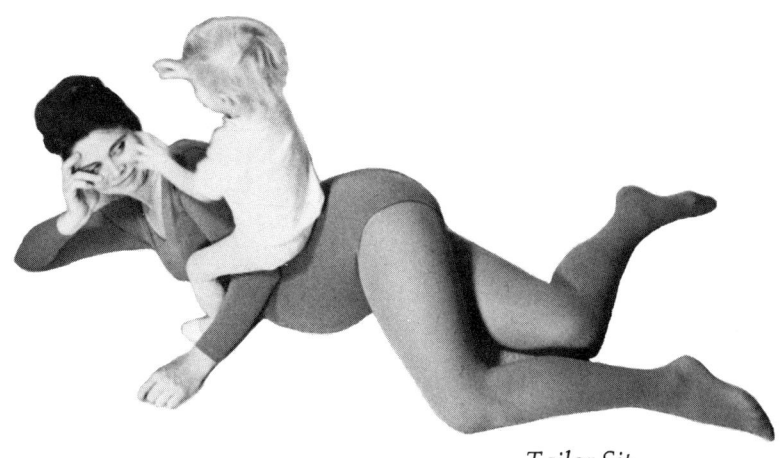

Tailor Sit
Pelvic Rock
Relaxation
Abdominal Breathing
Squat

As you begin Class One, your pregnancy is very exciting and almost unreal. It is so ever-present in your mind that it's hard to believe it doesn't "show" to anyone you pass on the street. You feel so new and different. You think about new philosophies of life. You become aware of the environment around you as totally changed. Some of the newness and change is somewhat unpleasant. Things bother you that have never bothered you before—the creak of the bathroom door can be screamingly irritating. Your husband's unexpected love pat makes you cry. ("It hurt," you say, wondering why you are crying.) You feel "left out" at work when you are not invited to join a group for lunch—a group that you never wanted to join in the past.

Are you nodding your head? Do you know what I'm saying? Perhaps you were the rare exception and escaped this normal experience of early pregnancy.

I wish that all of you could escape the nausea of pregnancy. It is the most unpleasant part of having babies! I was nauseous (rarely did I vomit). It disappeared around the fourth month but still I complain. To those of you who endure nine months of vomiting I offer condolences. Nausea in itself is not bad; it's that it goes on day after day, week after week, and becomes more a depression than an illness. That explains how you can feel better when there's a party to go to but feel "sick as a dog" Monday A.M. I compare the nausea of pregnancy to seasickness. It's not that you feel so horribly ill but rather that you can see no dry land on the horizon.

It does help the nausea if you will eat lots of protein to maintain a high blood sugar. Eating frequently helps, too. A bit of fruit every hour is what we suggest at the American Academy of Husband-Coached Childbirth. Fruit is less liable to turn you into a blimp than are candy, cake, and cookies. Remember, you are eating for two in quality, not quantity. Even with nausea and/or vomiting you must maintain a well-balanced diet. Eating many small meals may be the answer to making you feel better while ensuring your and the baby's good health. Instead of reaching for a cookie, have a small slice of whole wheat bread. Don't munch on a candy bar; chew on a crisp, juicy apple instead. Become aware of what you put into your body now that you are responsible for the health of two of you.

You have so many new things to think about with this new situation—your pregnancy. Perhaps you've never thought much about foods and now you find yourself checking on the number of grams of protein in what you eat. You must plan your home around a new body—perhaps paint the extra bedroom or even move to an apartment where babies are allowed. Sometimes it requires moving a two-year-old out of the crib. Your wardrobe has to be considered and a few changes made (your husband's summer sport shirts with a pair of tights make an inexpensive increase in your closet).

One of the biggest decisions you must make is choosing a doctor. It's best if you and your husband can have the first visit together. You will want to know his routine of prenatal care and you will especially want to know what type of preparation for childbirth he offers, what his feelings are on medications, what type of support he will offer you in labor, whether or not he expects your husband to stay with you, and, in general, his attitude to your needs and wishes regarding the childbirth experience. Your husband can be of much help in making your desires known to the doctor and in assessing the situation. In most cases, you'll have a choice of several doctors—so do a bit of "shopping," then choose the best. If you have only *one* choice of M.D., then proceed very slowly and cautiously, even deviously, to get your own way. As Dr. H. Ratner, on the Advisory Medical Board of La Leche League International, says of getting your ideas through to M.D.s, you must seduce them to your way of thinking, not attack them. Know what you want and expect to get it but don't be abusive about it!

By now you will have experienced the strange phenomena that your pregnancy creates in others. Everyone is an expert and has advice to offer. The mailman, the office boy, the boss, the shoe salesman, your parents, the lady next door, the grocery cart pusher behind you at the supermarket—all have tales to tell. Reactions vary from "How lovely" to "Poor little thing, you got caught," or even "There are enough children in the world already." You collect old wives' tales and folk medicine everywhere you go. You'll get some good advice, too, but sorting it all out is the problem.

Do not let your husband feel guilty about your bad days or your nausea. He did not do that to you! You became pregnant together. Hopefully, you and your husband can maintain good communication throughout this time in your pregnancy. It's vital to you both. Never have you needed a sounding board more and never have his needs for reassurance been greater. Let him know that you are normal and healthy and want to have this baby. A close, loving relationship is so important to the role of parenting. Sharing your love for each other with your baby increases the amount of love—it does not decrease it. It is an enrichment and a fulfillment which makes your relationship with each other bigger and wider as you expand to include another family member. But you are not sure of that yet and it's O.K. to be a bit worried about sharing your life with another person. The worry will be gone when you hold your baby in your arms.

Your sex life may change, too. Your poor husband should know that he is not being punished or rewarded (depending on which direction your needs take). Talk with him about the changes in you. You may not get to understand yourself any better, but at least friend husband will learn that you don't know what's going on any more than he does. I guess the most important thing for your marriage is to "keep talking," and listening, too.

Stop and think of all the variations in your life because you conceived. Loosen up, relax, take a deep breath, and stop being so hard on yourself. Accept your pregnancy and allow yourself *some* limitations.

Don't try to pretend that you are exactly the same person you were two or three months ago. At the same time, don't try to accept it all in one big swallow. It's always hard for the female; we have to accept motherhood in a matter of a week or two, whereas the father can take nine months to grasp his role. Every one of us has gone through the whole gamut of emotions. We each do it our own way.

Now let's get back to that initial response to your pregnant state —excitement! That seems to be the prevailing and overriding emotion that surpasses all the other reactions and keeps you going.

The first time we get together in Class One, we need to discuss what natural childbirth is. Most of you already have firm ideas about natural childbirth but once you commit yourself to it, you will need to be able to defend what you are doing. Many people will say, "You are so brave." I am not brave enough to have a baby any other way! How can anyone be brave enough to give up total responsibility for the birth of her baby? Yet for years it was accepted practice that the doctor would "take care of you." ("Leave it all to me, dearie.") It was a myth. No one can have your baby for you—and no one else can make it easy for you.

You must accept this as your responsibility. *You* will have this baby. *You* will prepare your body to give birth, and *you* will understand what is happening in your body to be able to work with the birth rather than against it. Birth is a natural process. There is a natural opening in your body which allows the birth of the baby. It is not surgery. We enjoy a society that takes the precaution of hospital deliveries so that most of the complications associated with childbirth can be safely cared for by medical expertise. But that does not mean that you should be subjected to medical methods when you can give birth with joy, love, and lots of plain, honest hard work. It may even be easy, but don't count on that!

Explain, when you are asked, that we are using educated childbirth rather than medicated childbirth. We are preparing very carefully so that you will understand what your body is doing as you give birth, and you will be able to work with the forces of birth. This makes for ease—not dis-ease. Pregnancy and birth are not abnormal, unnatural, diseased states of your life but, rather, normal and natural—and we hope to add the ease!

Natural childbirth has been around a long time and has many connotations in people's minds. Some consider it primitive—ours is educated. Some think it is an endurance test—ours is good preparation. Some think of it as training for the type of anesthesia your doctor will use—ours use absolutely no medication unless complications arise. Some think of it as a home delivery with no skilled medical person to "get in the way"—ours is a doctor-attended hospital birth with good support from the whole staff. Some think it is not making use of the medical expertise that has been developed over the years—ours is based on the newest scientific evidence that *any* anesthetic given prior to the birth of the baby does get into the baby's system—yes, even a local—and that any dosage which will be effective for the mother is a huge overdose for her infant.* You may even hear that natural childbirth is unsafe; yet the very basis for natural childbirth is the decreased risk from anesthesia for both mother and baby. It is the only safe way to protect the health of both. As a secondary benefit, it has turned out to be the most pleasant way to have a baby. Some may say that natural childbirth causes great guilt and disappointment in those who *do* require anesthesia —ours are satisfied parents who did their best. Certainly it's disappointing to have needed a Caesarean section or to have some complication requiring the use of forceps (therefore, anesthesia), or to have your doctor prescribe an anesthetic for medical reasons. As long as each woman is convinced that her doctor had her best interests in mind and that he did not "put one over on her," there is never a problem. It puts the burden on the doctor, then, to use anesthesia only when necessary, to reassure his patient of the need for anesthesia when used, and to make sure he has the complete trust of his patients. Surely that is not asking too much of our doctors! Natural childbirth is a practical approach to having a baby which trains the husband and wife for their roles in labor. The doctor supports the parents in labor and uses medical intervention only in those rare cases when it is necessary. All three work together as a team. The doctor is the expert, the father is the coach, and the mother does the work!

All this adds up to the fact that you will have nine months of explaining what you plan to do in the name of natural childbirth. There may even be some large gaps in definition between you and your doctor. Begin early to close them so that your labor can be as relaxed as possible. Husbands are essential in helping create a good communication with your doctor. Again I warn you, ask positively but do not demand, lest you nip all progress in the bud.

Old wives' tales can be a bother at the time of the first class, too.

* Bowes, Brackbill, Conway, and Steinschneider, *The Effects of Obstetric Medication on Fetus and Infant*, a monograph for the Society for Research in Child Development (University of Chicago Press, 1970).

With all that unsolicited advice you are getting, you don't know what to believe. "Never raise your hands over your head." "You mustn't hold in your tummy." "Take a long walk every day." "If you have heartburn, the baby will have lots of hair." "If you feel ugly and awkward, you'll have a girl." "If you feel pretty, you'll have a boy." "You must not paint while pregnant." "Don't climb stairs," and so on. If you feel troubled about whether or not they are nonsense, do ask your doctor. Remember, we are not very far out of the Victorian era, when pregnant females did not even go out in public. Some old wives' tales are based on shreds of outdated fact, but most of them you can ignore—all the ones I've listed you may surely ignore.

A word about asking your doctor questions. He is usually a very busy man and will be impatient with you if you seem to dilly-dally and want to chat. I have found it helpful if I have a businesslike list of questions for my visit to the doctor's office. (Don't overdo and have three pages full.) This facilitates things for both of you; the doctor knows he has answered your problems, and you go home with a good feeling of satisfaction. Monthly visits to your doctor are very important. So little seems to be accomplished that you may have the urge to skip a few months—but really, much information is recorded by the doctor. Small changes in you, especially in blood pressure, rapid weight gain, and swelling, need to be noted so your doctor will be able to prevent possible problems. There are large volumes of statistics which prove the chances of health and life of mothers and babies are vastly improved with good prenatal care. Allow the medical professionals to use their skill in preventing disease rather than waiting until it may be too late for a cure!

You will attend Class One soon after your initial visit to your doctor, which may be in your second or third month. By the time you are three months pregnant your baby weighs about one ounce. The baby has definitely become a boy or a girl by now, but you are not let in on the secret. Arms and legs begin to move. His head is developed, with eyes, ears, nose, and mouth. The bones have begun to form in his body. The whole sac in which the baby grows is about the size of a goose egg.

Now let's talk about the exercises. They are not calisthenics. In most cases, they are postures and not exercises at all—but exercise is an easy word to use. On the schedule cards we mail to our class members we call them Rock and Relax, rather than exercise, classes. This is a very relaxed form of exercise. You do not compete with anyone—you do the best *you* can. Most of our postures are designed to be used around the home in your everyday activities. Many can be done anywhere you work but all can easily be fit in if you work at home all day. Some are to be used for your pregnancy, some prepare you for labor, but many are to be maintained for the rest of your life. Do not make yourself stiff and sore by overusing your muscles at first. Begin slowly and increase gradually and you will have pleasant results. We like to have one month between classes, which gives you enough time to work to proficiency on what you've learned before we go on to some more. Each class will review and check you on previous exercises to make sure it is all clear. You will be the judge of how many times you should do each posture. We give you guidelines in many cases—but remember that you are the one who will have the baby. If your muscles are not ready for labor, who is to blame? If you haven't practiced enough on your abdominal breathing, it's very hard to learn while in labor. In most cases, your husband, the labor coach, will be very hard on you and insist on a good nine months of training. It will be to your benefit if he helps you that way.

Let's begin with our first "exercise"—tailor sitting.

Tailor Sit

Never stand when you can sit; and when you sit, tailor sit!

Why? Because tailor sitting is comfortable. Children and more "natural" cultures use this position without teaching.

Sitting tailor fashion, with your elbows on your knees, tilts the heavy uterus forward, away from your back and up and out of the pelvis. This teeter-totter effect, with the uterus tilted over the front of the pelvic bone, allows release of pressure and, therefore, good circulation of blood to the pelvic area, to kidneys, vagina, and legs.

Tailor sitting keeps you from sitting in a chair in the usual manner, leaning back and allowing backward tilt of the uterus, which puts pressure on blood vessels supplying the kidneys and legs, thereby reducing circulation. Crossing your knees further aggravates the problem and reduces circulation to the vagina.

Tailor sitting stretches and makes flexible the muscles of your bottom and the inner aspects of your thighs, enabling you to put your legs farther apart in second-stage labor, which will be helpful. It may sound ridiculous, but the effect of increased light and air to your perineum is a healthy extra as it may help prevent vaginal yeast infections (monilia).

HOW Sit on the floor or any firm surface. Cross your ankles and bring them close to your body with knees wide apart. (You may lean back slightly to reduce the weight on your ankles.) This is not an exercise, but rather a posture.

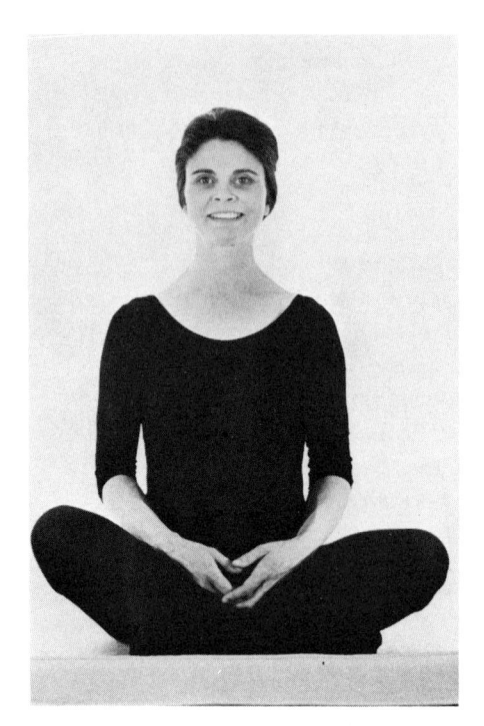

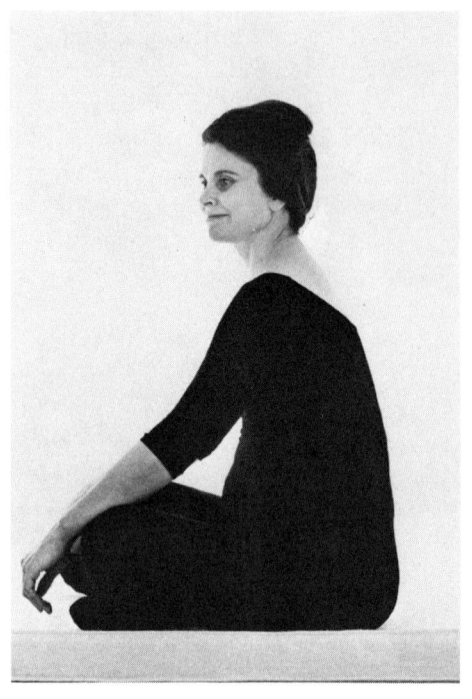

Variations. You may use variations to keep comfortable while sitting for longer periods. As one position becomes crampy, change to a variation:

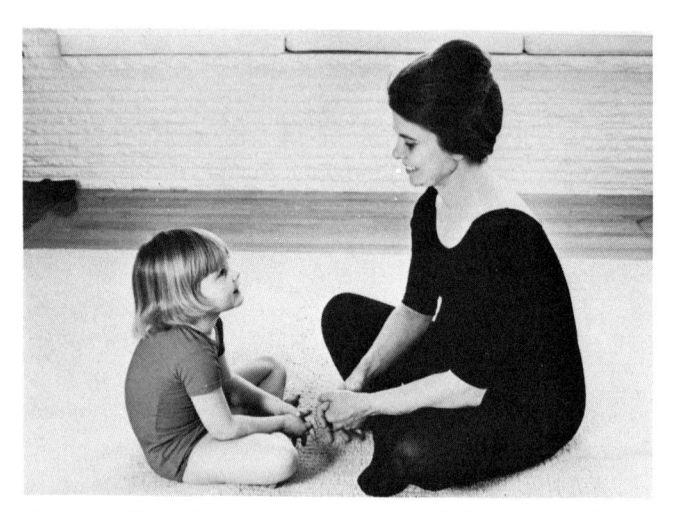

- Ankles in a "nearly lotus" position, with feet on the floor rather than on your thighs.

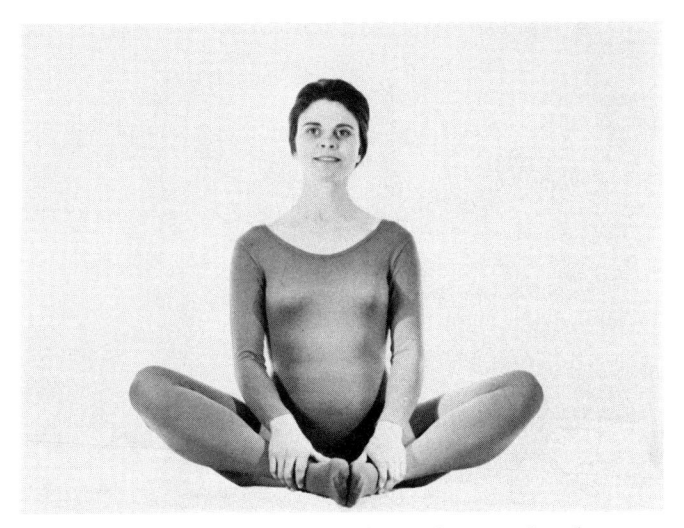

- Soles of feet together, with knees bent and wide apart.

Do not sit in any one position for long periods of time or your legs will go to sleep from lack of good circulation. Even if you sit in a chair, you don't punish yourself by never moving! Most of us find this tailor sitting position easy from all our activities in normal life, but if it is difficult for you, rest your elbows on your knees with slight pressure. Don't force your knees to the floor. That is not necessary and may be painful. After a few weeks you'll be comfortable for longer periods and your knees will come closer to the floor. Your knees may never touch the floor, since individuals differ. If you are very limber and your knees do fall apart to touch the floor, this position will be very easy for you to use. You are ahead of most of us in preparation for childbirth!

There are other problems than loose muscles that can keep you from doing tailor sitting, I discovered. One evening when I was teaching a class to tailor sit, we had a guest who had come with her friend. She participated in the class with enthusiasm until I had explained the tailor sit position and asked everyone to use it. Our guest refused. She had been brought up in a home and a country (Mexico) where young ladies conducted themselves in a formal way and sitting cross-legged on the floor did not fit into her life style at all. I encouraged her, and I encourage you, to try the loose, easy, relaxed informality that suits our day and age and makes pregnancy so much easier.

WHERE Always choose a hard, level surface so that your hips and feet are on the same plane.

WHEN Anytime you can sit down! For example: Diapering the baby, reading to the children or yourself, doing knitting, needlework, or whatever handicrafts you enjoy. Cleaning drawers or lower cupboards (take the drawer out of the chest and put it on the floor). Riding in a car,

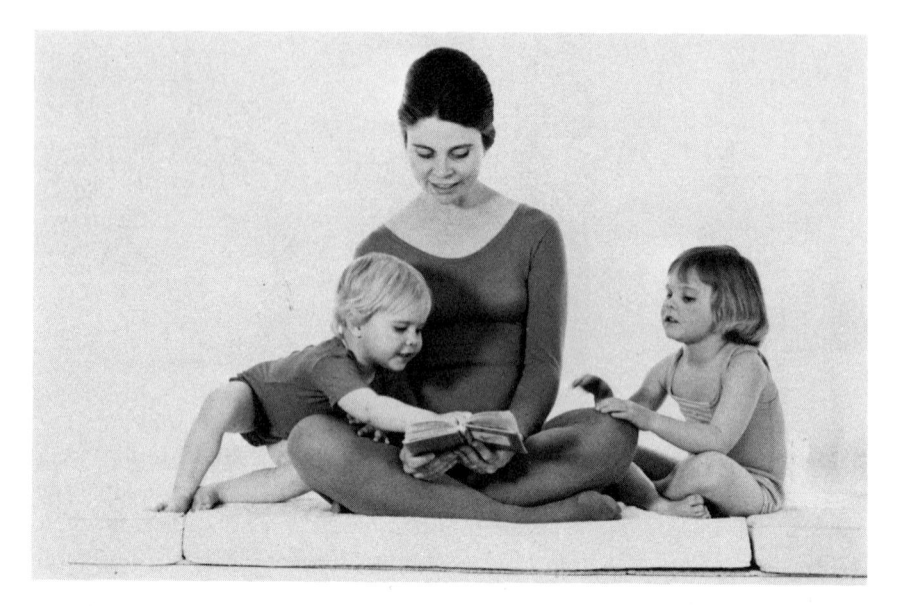

watching television, writing letters, watching drive-in movies, eating dinner at a coffee table, sitting on the floor, usually in your own home. Playing cards or any games when you can sit on the floor instead of in a chair. Wouldn't your bridge club all benefit? Conversation—sit on the floor, not on the sofa. With children, everything you do. You will be on their level as you dress, feed, cuddle, hug, listen, talk, play, fix a hurt, pick up toys—the list is twenty-four hours long! You can sit this way in many chairs, such as ordinary hard kitchen or dining chairs (though you may need a pad for your ankles).

One of my special contributions to young mothers is to free them from standing long hours at the ironing board. That is not to say I relieve you of your ironing (though a lovely "new baby" gift is a month's ironing done by a friend). If you can afford to pay a nonpregnant ironing lady, do it by all means. However, my solution is to free you from standing by insisting that you *sit* at the ironing board. The long hours can be avoided by doing a bit of ironing now and then or some each day. When you iron, pull the ironing board up to a piano bench, sofa, or bed where you can tailor sit and where there is room to sort and to place pieces as they are finished. If you've ironed long enough for your legs to feel cramped, it's time to put some pieces away and ready some more to iron. My little girls, when they play-iron, sit like queens and don't know that some people stand or walk around the ironing board to do the same work. It is a legacy that you'll pass to your daughters—or maybe your sons, the way our society is changing. Cut down on your ironing by reading the labels on children's clothes before buying. Buy only the truly non-iron type of wash-and-wear.

Sit in the tailor position for short periods or as long as it is comfortable. One woman told me in a class that she was having trouble with this posture. She claimed that it caused her legs to fall asleep. I checked her position and it was perfect. I reviewed some minor variations and she knew them all. But she insisted that it was very uncomfortable for her to sit in the tailor position. We talked about where and when she was sitting this way and it all sounded normal. Since tailor sitting is an uncomplicated position, there had to be a reason for her discomfort. I began cross-examining her. It seemed she was having the most trouble with her legs falling asleep during TV watching. I was ready to give up and tell her to keep trying and gradually her legs would become more used to it, when I had a flash thought. I had not asked how many minutes of TV she watched without moving. Sure enough, her idea of a reasonable amount of time was not the amount that her legs could tolerate. She was sitting through a TV movie, two hours, without getting up and moving around. A superhuman effort.

My point is that you must exercise a certain amount of good sense in how you use a posture or exercise. Do them as often and as long as you like. But do be kind to yourself and work up gradually to your optimum.

If tailor sitting is easy for you, it will be used for a more extended period of time than if you find it difficult. However, it should be used with the idea that you are not trying to set a new record. Make it a part of your life, a useful and comfortable addition to your way of doing things which will also contribute to your health. Think of tailor sitting as your friend, not as an enemy.

Pelvic Rock

We imitate animals in natural childbirth. In the pelvic rock, we imitate four-footed animals in posture and does it feel good! Standing erect causes the uterus, as it becomes heavier and heavier with pregnancy, to push lower and more tightly into the pelvis. This compresses the blood vessels and interferes with circulation to the uterus, legs, and kidneys. The heavy uterus also stretches supportive ligaments that are attached in the small of the back at roughly the same position as in four-footed mammals. The pressure and the weight cause the pregnant female to "give in" to the uterus, letting it fall forward and sway her back. Backache and "pressure" pains are the result. Pelvic rocking on hands and knees allows the uterus to fall forward, releasing the pressure in the pelvis and causing no discomfort in the spine because of the all-fours position. In this posture, your spine is a bridge supported on either end by arms and legs, whereas in a standing position your spine is an upright pole supporting you. A bridge can be sturdy with a sway in it, but get out of the way of a swaying pole!

What does pelvic rocking do for you? There is a long list of benefits, but the basic results are that you will look and feel better. This is an exercise to help you during pregnancy rather than in labor. It strengthens muscles in your back and abdomen and therefore makes it easier for you to carry the baby in your uterus.

Pelvic rocking improves your posture for the rest of your life. (This *is* a lifetime exercise.) A straight spine makes you feel and look better whether you are pregnant or not. Pelvic rocking strengthens your back muscles. The muscles along your spine need to be very strong to be able to maintain a straight spine while a heavy uterus is attached to it.

Pelvic rocking strengthens abdominal muscles to support the uterus, and what a difference in the figure immediately postpartum—after birth. Your tummy will be flatter than ever before. You may even reduce the size and flabbiness of your hips and thighs. You should never need a girdle again—oh, blessed relief! Nor will you look as though you need one.

Pelvic rocking will help prevent varicose veins by increasing circulation to pelvis and legs. Relieving the pressure of the uterus in the pelvis will relieve pressure on the blood vessels there. Any mild exercise improves circulation, so by pelvic rocking you are restoring good circulation to your pelvis and legs. The relief of pelvic pressure and increased circulation helps prevent hemorrhoids, too.

Pelvic rocking increases mobility of the pelvis, which may help in labor as you push the baby through the birth canal.

Pelvic rocking will definitely help relieve tensions and relax you in preparation for bed at night. (Do extra when you are "too tired to do *any.*")

HOW Get on the floor in an "all-fours" position, making sure that you form a box, with your knees and hips in a line and your wrists and shoulders also perpendicular to the floor. Knees may be comfortably apart.

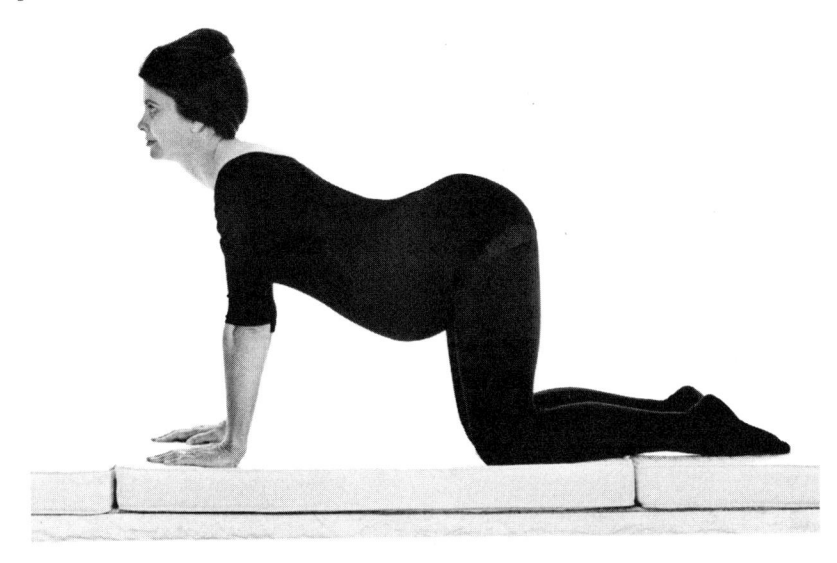

1. Lower your abdomen toward the floor until you look like a "sway-back horse."

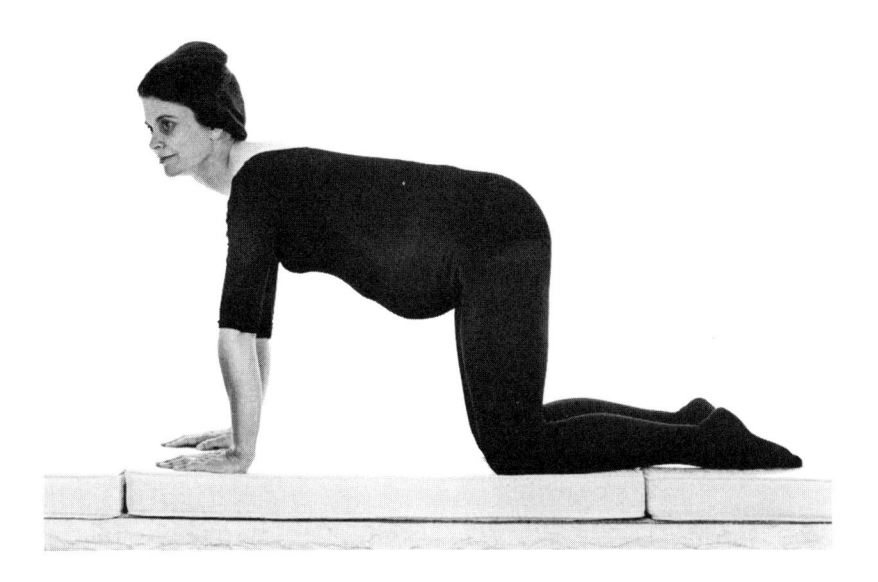

2. Lift your lower back until your back is parallel with the floor.
3. Tighten buttocks. This raises the back slightly and tightens the abdomen.
4. Slowly return to the "sway-back" first position with control.
5. Repeat movements 2 through 4.

This must be done rhythmically, with as much control lowering as raising the back. It should be done slowly, the whole movement taking about five to seven seconds. Do not move your shoulders and upper back. This exercise is for the lower back and pelvis and we ignore the upper back completely. Do not move your arms either.

Watching yourself in a mirror while doing this exercise will help you do the movements. If you do not have a full-length mirror, try putting a light on the floor to cast your shadow on the wall.

If you develop a pain or a "stitch" in your side as when running, it is a result of dropping your abdomen too quickly or too low. Use more control and there will be only comfort, never discomfort.

WHERE This is very hard to combine with any routine chore unless you are beautifully uninhibited, as was my first natural childbirth teacher, Peggy Rice. At a cocktail party one evening where everyone was rather formal, pregnant Peggy felt a nagging backache. She put her drink down and, in her long dress, got on the floor on all fours and began pelvic rocking, chatting all the while to a very startled male guest.

If you can't emulate Peggy, you will have to get off by yourself several times during the day to do enough pelvic rocks to keep you comfortable. For those of you working outside your homes through a pregnancy, you might find a ladies' lounge or an unused conference room, a supply room—anyplace where you can get on all fours and do pelvic rocks to relieve the tension in your back. The first thing you should do as you walk into your home after work is to get down on your knees—double meaning intended! If your husband is waiting impatiently for dinner, take time to fix him his favorite drink first, then the two of you can visit while you relax your uterus and back.

WHEN Do last thing before bed—that is very important. Do eighty before bed, with a rest in between! Do at intervals during the day. For example: midmorning, midafternoon, and early evening, forty each time, then eighty at bedtime, too. If this is your first pregnancy, you may not feel the need of the daytime pelvic rocks until your uterus has grown big enough to make you aware of a bit of pressure. If you have already had a child, you'll want to pelvic rock all day long because it feels so good.

Rest position during pelvic rock. If your arms become tired before finishing the required eighty at bedtime, you may use this posture for a few minutes, then continue with pelvic rocking. Dr. Bradley calls this the "froggy" position.

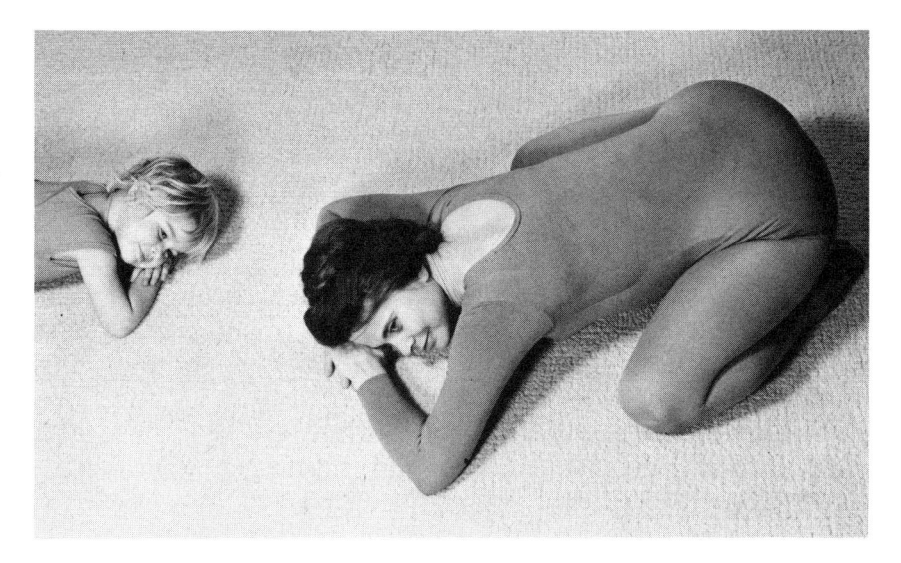

1. Spread knees a bit farther apart and have toes pointing straight back.
2. Sit on your heels and let your torso lean forward toward the floor so that your arms and head can rest on the floor. If this is not comfortable (you need stretchy or very loose clothing), use a pillow under your chest and head.
3. Relax.

Relaxation

Relaxation is a state of physical passivity but mental activity. In other words, you work hard with your mind to keep your body quiet! It is very different from actual sleep, when our minds probably fall asleep before our bodies relax. Relaxing takes mental discipline, especially while the uterus is in hard contraction. During relaxation as used in labor, there is absolutely no sleepiness involved, but rather a very heightened awareness and complete control over oneself. You may even think of yourself as "working hard" at relaxing. Remember, it is very passive work physically but hard work mentally.

The meaning of the word "relaxation" as we will use it may be very different from your past experience. It will be a skill that you will find useful for the rest of your life. I think it is a shame that we spend *no* time in schools teaching children consciously to relax. It is a much needed ability throughout life.

Relaxation must be considered the most important factor in an enjoyable childbirth experience. Relaxing is in fact the crux of natural childbirth. The only help you can give the uterus with its work in first stage is to "let it be." Do not interfere. To do this requires great concentration on relaxing because the uterus contracts to a hard knot. It is a sensation that you can ease your body through if you're relaxed, but what a difference if you are tense! The uterine contraction has many times greater intensity when the muscles surrounding it are also tense.

The theory of why relaxation makes your contractions feel better I will leave to Dr. Bradley to explain.* I've done it five times in childbirth and know that it is so—and each one of you may try it for herself. It is a very easy theory to prove in labor.

Our second labor began, as I've told you, at a La Leche meeting at Mary Ann Kerwin's. I called Richard to come for me so we could go on to the hospital from there. Things were going well. I was relaxed on a sofa, feeling as though we had lots of time, so Richard and Tom Kerwin had some cake and coffee, left from the meeting refreshments. There was much fun and laughing, the four of us being rather excited. It was a joke in the middle of a contraction that changed my attitude. When I tried to laugh, I realized that my contractions were very strong and hard and we'd better not dawdle too long. Relaxing too well can fool you! I did have enough time, however.

The point of this incident is that you may feel so comfortable you'll not know that your relaxing is responsible for your comfort and that your labor is actually hard. Getting "caught" in the bathroom, laughing, coughing, or trying to be polite and answer a nurse—any activity in the middle of a contraction will prove to you by contrast that relaxation works.

Just remember that any part of your body in tension is going to add tension to the uterine contraction. It also detracts from the uterus's efficiency. Stay out of the way and let the uterus do its work. You'll feel better and the labor will not be slowed down.

* See *Husband-Coached Childbirth.*

HOW *Classic Position.* Lie on your side on a firm padded surface with one arm under and behind you, the other bent in front of your face. Both legs are bent at the knee, the upper one pulled forward to help support the weight of your body away from the baby.

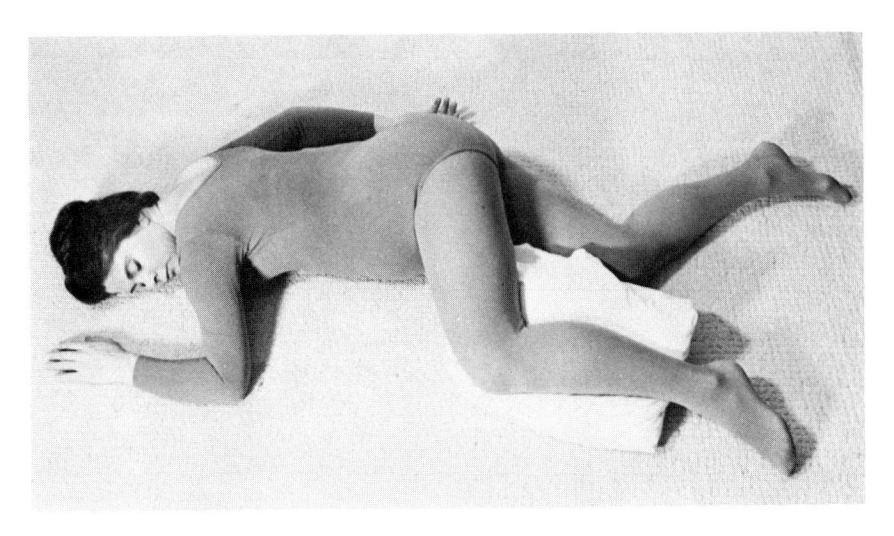

Pillows may be used wherever necessary to make you more comfortable—under your knee (as shown), or under the head and chest to help hold your weight off the lower shoulder.

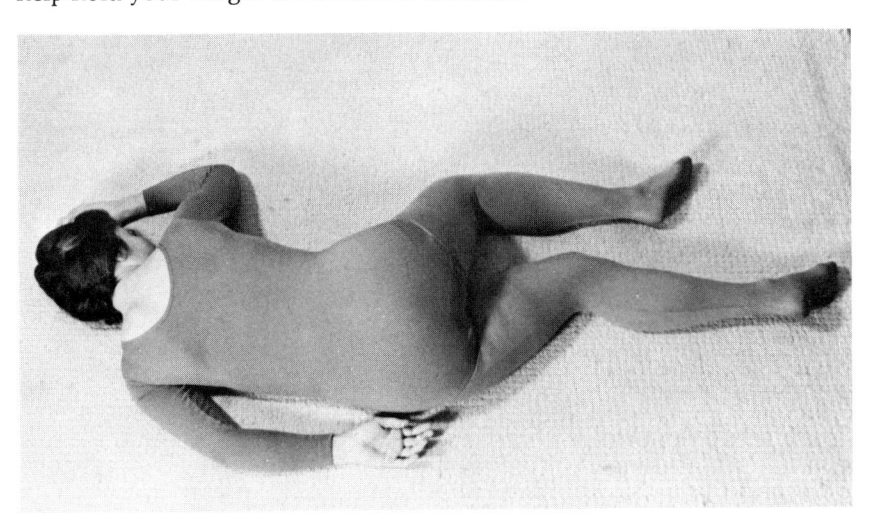

Variation of Classic Position. Your arms may be more comfortable in front, but avoid putting one arm on top of the other or holding your head on your arms, which creates a point of tension.

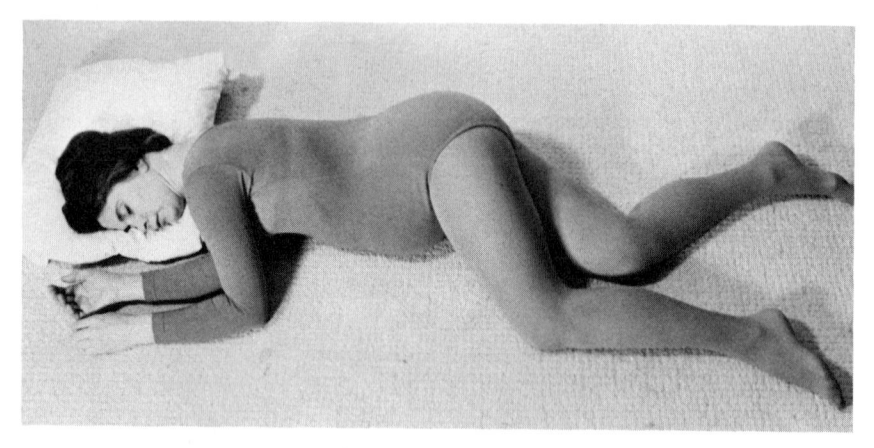

Contour Position. Each part of the body is supported with pillows to prevent tension. This position may be useful during transition.

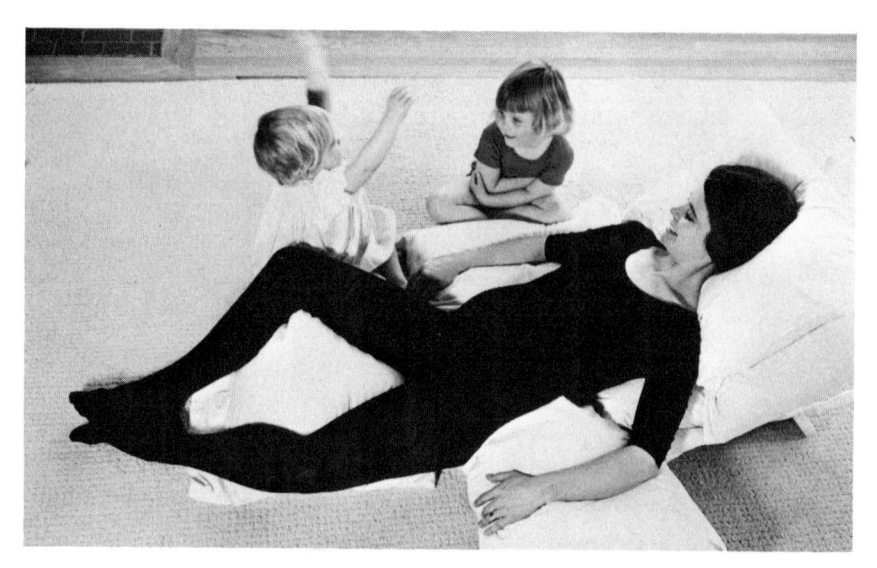

To prepare for relaxation, especially during labor, keep in mind these necessary conditions:

1. The proper atmosphere includes absence of strangers, darkness, solitude, and quiet; a quiet, restful room with as little unexpected noise or commotion as possible. Avoid a glaring light, but a soft, dull light will aid your efforts to relax.

2. Use a comfortable position, as shown. This basic position varies some with each individual, but whatever your position, each joint should be slightly bent, not straight or fully flexed. Position your body and use pillows to help you become comfortable, with all tension relieved. When you are in labor, the hospital bed will adjust to help with your positioning. Do not let any one part of the body bear the weight of any other part of the body—in other words, don't have your head resting on your arm, or one leg on the other.

3. Control your breathing. Use slow, steady, and relaxed abdominal breathing. We will discuss this technique fully later on. See pages 36–39.

4. Complete concentration and attention to what you are doing is imperative. Closing your eyes helps you control your environment. You shut it out!

Now, assuming the classic position, get yourself as comfortable and relaxed as you can. If you then read the poem I've written (see pages 34–35), you should be able to relax even more. You'll soon observe how you respond to different words and phrases, and if necessary begin to think creatively about what other words or routines might be better for you. If you wish to begin at the toes and work up the body, that is as good as using the baby as the focal point, as I have done. You may prefer to use a "total body" idea of relaxing and not go to the progressive method at all. Perhaps you will do best with "pleasant thought" or meditative relaxing.

My husband with his gift of words is marvelous at relaxing me. I did not have to teach him how; he knew how to relax himself. Not all people are alike and many of you will benefit in labor if you teach your husband to relax now. Prove to him how relaxing it is to speak softly and lovingly. Show him how hard it is to keep tension in his face when you are offering suggestions of a relaxed face. Demonstrate how a bad position hinders his relaxing. Test out words and touching to see how he responds. When he has learned to relax, he will be better able to help you relax.

One couple had spent time together working and planning for the labor. He had given careful thought to helping his wife relax and when the time came for the real thing, they did very well. During one of the contractions, the father-to-be became either tired or excited (probably both) and as part of the relaxing monologue said, "Now, relax your hair." That was the end of relaxation with that contraction, as she burst into giggles. He used more sensible suggestions for relaxing during the remainder of their labor.

I offer what we have used effectively in class for years as a way of easily teaching others to relax—often a very new skill for many people in our fast-living society. So begin with this and then progress to your own variation. Even if you continue to use my words, you will place your own meaning on them. Relaxing is so personal that I can only teach it the way I feel it. Try to tune in with me and let it work for you.

Now have your husband read (croon) this to you slowly, quietly as a poem or a lullaby, giving time for it to take effect:

> *Let your whole being*
> *sink slowly, slowly, slowly.*
> *Feel your muscles*
> *becoming limp and loose and comfortable.*
> *Drifting or floating,*
> *relaxed and comfortable,*
> *warmth and heaviness spread through your body.*
> *The baby in your uterus*
> *is warm and heavy.*
> *Feel warmth and heaviness*
> *spreading from the baby to your abdomen, hips,*
> *thighs, knees, lower legs, ankles,*
> *feet, and toes.*
> *Slowly, the lower half of you is*
> *loose and limp,*
> *warm and heavy.*
>
> *The upper half of you awaits its turn.*
> *Slowly release, let go,*
> *warm and heavy,*
> *limp and loose.*
> *Let every cell absorb and enjoy,*
> *spreading up back and front,*
> *chest and shoulders.*
> *Arms and fingers let go.*

*As your neck releases tension,
your head slowly shifts and becomes
more and more relaxed.
Nearer and nearer that comfortable state of
relaxation.*

*Erase the worries from your brow,
eyes loose but closed.
Eyes and all around eyes
limp and loose.
Cheeks loosen and droop,
jaw drops.
Tongue is loose in your mouth,
lips part slightly.
Warm, heavy, and comfortable.*

*Deep, slow, heavy breathing.
Breathe in and out slowly,
abdomen up and down slowly.
Limp and loose,
warm and heavy,
comfortably relaxed.*

*In your mind's eye
hold a softly purring kitten in your lap
while sunshine warms you both.
Listen to the laughter of children
sledding on a crisp sparkly snowy hill.
Ride a bicycle on a lazy autumn afternoon,
hair blowing in the wind.
Sit before a roaring, snapping fire
with a crisp apple ready to eat.
Watch a robin build her nest,
weaving string and straw with precision.
Lie on the warm sand, you and your love,
while the waves roll up on the beach.*

*Limp and loose,
warm and heavy,
comfortably relaxed.*

WHERE AND WHEN You will relax completely and breathe abdominally during each contraction in the first stage of labor—in between contractions you will not need to relax. Preparing for labor will take much practice, so relax whenever you can lie down for a nap and every night as you go to bed. It takes only minutes and will help you relax for sleep. One good way to test yourself is to spend two minutes on the floor of your living room (or wherever you have a rug on the floor) at the busiest time of your day. 10 A.M., maybe? You may have a toddler pulling at your eyelids and asking, "Why sleep, Mommy?" but that is very good preparation for labor, when you must ignore your environment and concentrate on yourself. As I was getting ready to go to the hospital in my third labor, our two-year-old, Claryss Nan, did, as I have told you, try to open my eyes as I relaxed. So I mean what I say! Explain to your wee ones what you are doing and why; have them relax with you if they will. Set your timer for two minutes and relax. Put up with the crawling over you, the riding on your back, the fight in the next room, whatever. Labor may even seem easy by comparison! If you have a tendency to fall asleep and sleep for hours, despite what is going on around you, better set an alarm, or ask a neighbor to telephone you at an appointed time. Falling asleep is not good relaxing practice, however. You have stopped concentrating on your relaxation or you'd never fall asleep. So stay awake and think hard about relaxing.

You can relax at other times, too, of course. I do think it best to lie down, but sometimes you could sit in a chair and try to loosen your body as much as possible. Any efforts to relax will help you become better at it.

Abdominal Breathing

During the first stage of labor, with each contraction you will breathe with your abdomen and relax completely. Between contractions you may do what you feel like doing and breathe however you wish. Abdominal breathing and relaxation are a team. You do them better together than you are able to do each separately. Your ability to do both will increase with practice, so the amount of time you spend at it beforehand will pay great dividends during labor.

We have already discussed relaxation and referred to abdominal breathing. Now we will learn the basics of abdominal breathing and, from then on, you should do the two together.

When you breathe abdominally, you have the feeling that great amounts of air are being pulled into your abdominal cavity. This is impossible, of course. What is happening is that the diaphragm is pulling down into the abdomen so that the lungs can expand fully. The diaphragm is a muscle which acts as a bellows. It pulls down and air is sucked into the lungs. It pushes up and the lungs are emptied. Naturally, the bigger the amounts of air you take into your lungs, the slower your breathing will be and the higher your abdominal wall will rise.

When you inhale, your abdomen rises—as you exhale, it lowers. The breathing must be very slow and full. Give plenty of time for each part of the breath.

Since your body will be working very hard during labor, you will require great quantities of oxygen to fulfill your needs. At the same time, you must be totally relaxed for your labor to progress smoothly and easily. I do not recommend that you do this, but if you ran around the outside of your house, then put yourself into a relaxation position and practiced abdominal breathing, you would get the feeling of the kind of breathing required during labor. You would also notice that you needed your mouth open to get enough breath. Your muscles must be relaxed but your body is working hard and therefore requires big puffy breaths. So when we say, "Relax and breathe slowly and deeply," the effect in practice will be different from the real thing in labor.

Raising the abdominal wall as high as possible is important in labor for another reason. The uterus, as it tightens with a contraction, will bulge. This pushes it against the abdominal wall. Now, if your abdominal muscles are relaxed and being raised slowly with abdominal breathing, there will be minimal discomfort when the contracting, bulging uterus pushes against the abdominal wall. Pull tight on the abdominal muscles and see the tension created between two hard, contracted muscles—the uterus and the abdomen. (Don't do it on purpose, unless you don't believe me!)

So relaxing with abdominal breathing keeps the abdominal muscles soft and relaxed and slowly pushed away from the contracting uterus by your big oxygen-laden inhalation. During exhalation, the abdominal wall (indeed, the whole body) remains relaxed to avoid interference with the work of the contracting uterus.

It is so simple and makes such good sense! We are simply trying to let the uterus do its work by staying out of its way. At the same time, we must supply it with necessary materials. Deep breathing will supply the necessary amounts of oxygen to the blood. A good position allows adequate circulation to the uterus so the blood supply reaches it. The side-lying position best serves this need. However, the contour position is a possible variation, if necessary. Remember that lots of stretching and moving about between contractions will help keep you comfortable.

To sum up, abdominal breathing is necessary, first, because you need the large amount of oxygen that this type of deep breathing will allow. Ordinary breathing, usually much more shallow, cannot easily serve

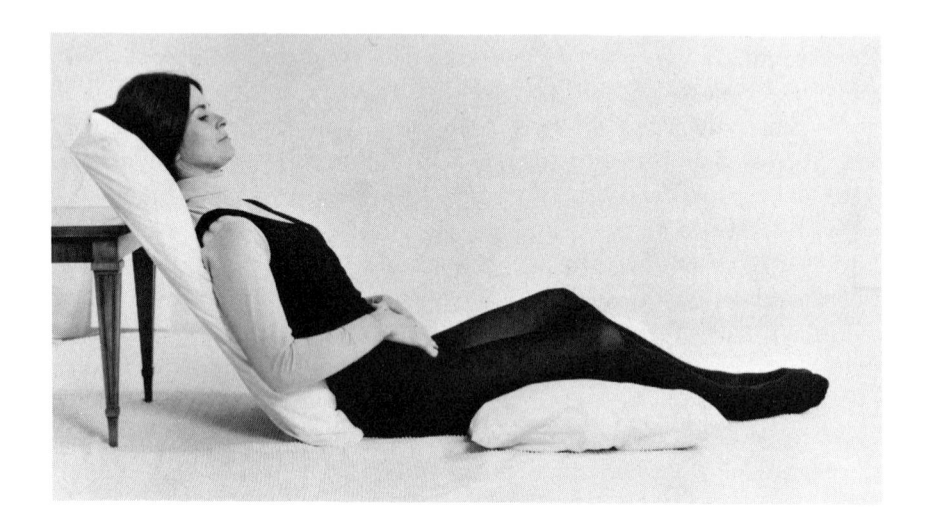

the great oxygen needs of the laboring body. Secondly, you can relax much better if you breathe in this manner, and only with relaxation will you be comfortable during first-stage labor. Thirdly, the control used in the breathing helps give you the mastery of your body required to "ride" with each contraction of the uterus. You are the director of this show!

HOW

1. Lie in a contour position with knees raised to lessen the tension of the abdominal muscles. (This position is for learning how, more than for labor. As soon as you have learned the technique, you may practice on your side in a relaxed position.)
2. Put hands low on abdomen so that you can feel the suprapubic bone. This guides you to take a deeper breath than if your hands are higher up on the abdomen.
3. Open your mouth and take a deep breath. Let the breath push your abdomen (and hands) up.
4. Let breath out and hands and abdomen go down again.

5. Repeat and practice for about two minutes.
6. Now put one hand up on your chest. There should be no chest movement as you continue to breath abdominally.

Stop and rest! Now continue, and try to make each breath as long in duration as is comfortable. Try to "fill your abdomen up" with air. Notice the difference between letting the breath push your abdomen up and having the muscles lift your abdomen. You *must not* tense your muscles. For you to be comfortable in labor, your abdominal wall must remain relaxed while the uterus is contracting. Sometimes this can be a confusing thing but your husband will be able to feel the difference with his hand and can coach you to know when you are doing well. Practice together now so that you'll be a good team when labor begins. He could read Dr. Bradley's *Husband-Coached Childbirth*, pages 60–62, to aid him in his understanding of the husband's role.

WHERE Where do you practice? In bed as you lie down for an afternoon rest, and when you are ready for sleep at night. Do several minutes of concentrated relaxation with abdominal breathing each time.

Begin to use abdominal breathing during the day as you think of it. As you first learn this type of breathing, you may despair that it will ever become easy. It quickly becomes a comfortable way of breathing, though, and by the time you go into labor, it should come very naturally. The more you practice, the easier your first stage of labor will be. When your labor reaches an intensity that demands your assistance, start relaxing and abdominal breathing with each contraction until the first stage of labor is completed and you are ready to begin pushing.

WHEN *During pregnancy.* Practice often during pregnancy—at least three times each day—taking several breaths. Consider two minutes a good amount of time for a practice contraction, although a contraction would not likely be this long—one minute to one and one-half minutes is more likely, even at transition (end of the first stage).

You will soon learn to breathe abdominally in other positions so that you can practice it all day long. Practice it while lying in a contour position only until you know for sure how to do it, then use the side-lying relaxation position.

In labor. With each contraction, relax completely and take deep, slow, full abdominal breaths.

Squat

This is not a ladylike posture, so think of it as "motherlike." It is important, so use it proudly.

The squat is the position you will assume to give birth. It opens the "baby door," for the pelvis is pulled as wide open as it can get. So get busy and limber up those squatting muscles! Many a mother, alas, has been instructed or forced to "hold her legs together" until the doctor arrived, to keep her baby from being born. This is effective in preventing birth—painfully. Therefore, the opposite holds true for hastening birth. The wider apart you hold your legs, the sooner the baby can be born—joyfully.

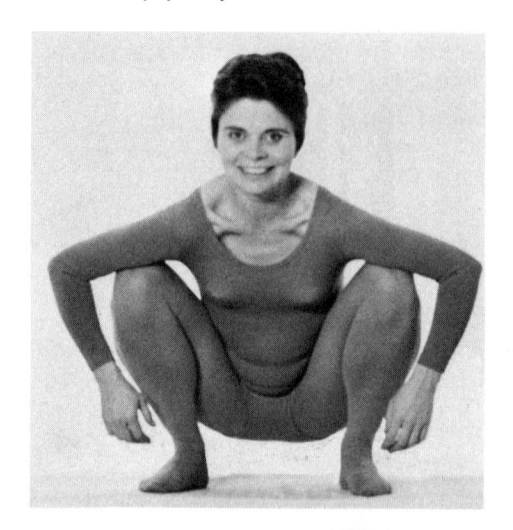

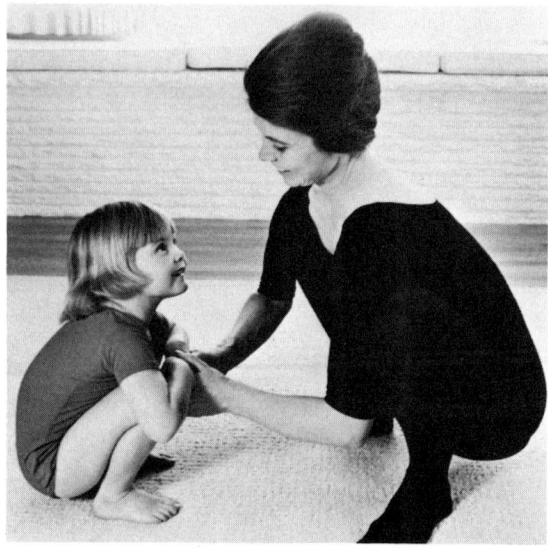

As I have mentioned, even the light and air admitted to this region of your body is healthful in preventing yeast infection (monilia), since yeast requires darkness and lack of oxygen to grow.

Squatting develops better circulation in the perineal area, which leads to better muscle tone and healthier tissue. By squatting you are preparing the perineum to stretch better to allow the birth of the baby. If an episiotomy—cutting of the perineum to facilitate the baby's passage—is necessary, healing is much faster and easier.

HOW Bend your knees into a squatting position, keeping heels on the floor and toes straight ahead. Keep weight on the outer edges of your feet as much as possible. With your knees wide apart, place your arms between them.

Use this position only as long as it is comfortable—actually, very short times. Even if you can stay in the squat position for a longer time, be careful, as you may feel "fused" into a squat position before you know it.

If you cannot balance and keep falling into a sitting position, hold on to a heavy object such as the bottom of a chest of drawers, a bed leg, the lower cupboards in the kitchen, the bottom of a closed door—anything that will support you and yet keep your hands low enough to maintain a proper squat position. It will help you if your clothes are loose or stretchy.

Getting up from a squat. To come up again, push tailbone toward ceiling as legs straighten, then raise upper portion of body upright. This helps tilt the heavy uterus up and out of the pelvis. It is a pelvic rock.

WHERE AND WHEN Squat anytime you find it necessary to reach low: getting into lower cupboards, gardening, picking up laundry or light objects, scrubbing floors, caring for children, changing diapers, tying shoes, loving, hugging, or talking to a child, helping dress, buttoning, showing things, explaining, etc. However, you must *not* lift any weight from a squat position.

You may have to restrict this position to times and places when you are alone—or risk being laughed at. I vividly recall using this posture as a matter of habit when I was ten years old, until my friends embarrassed me by laughing at my lack of sophistication. When I was in college, however, it became fashionable to squat—it was called "hunkering." You may or may not be acceptable when you use this posture, so you must have conviction about how good it is for you.

42 EXERCISES FOR TRUE NATURAL CHILDBIRTH

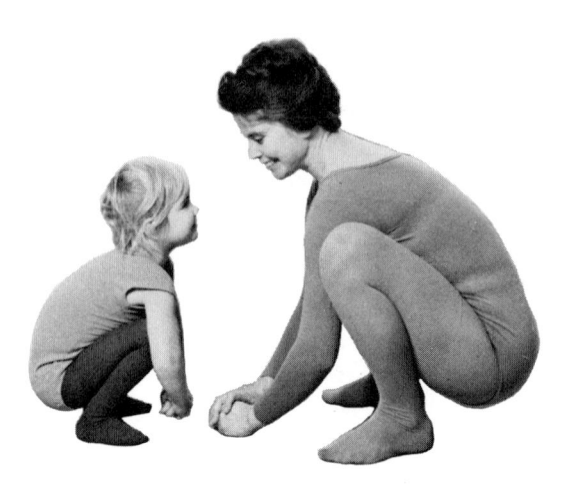

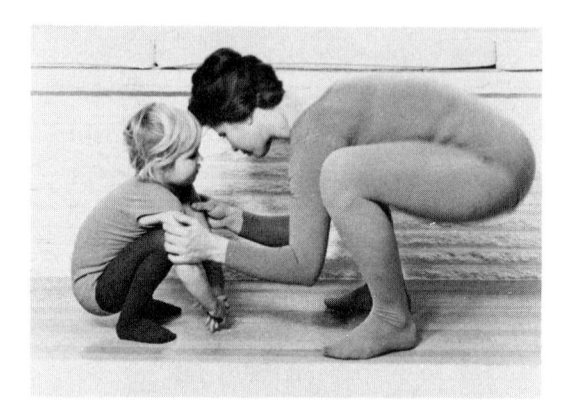

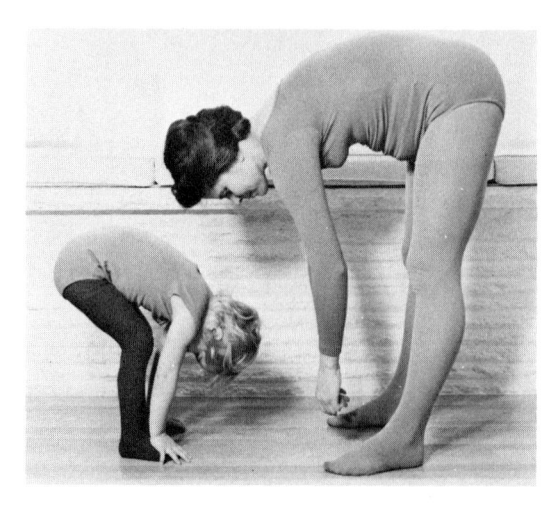

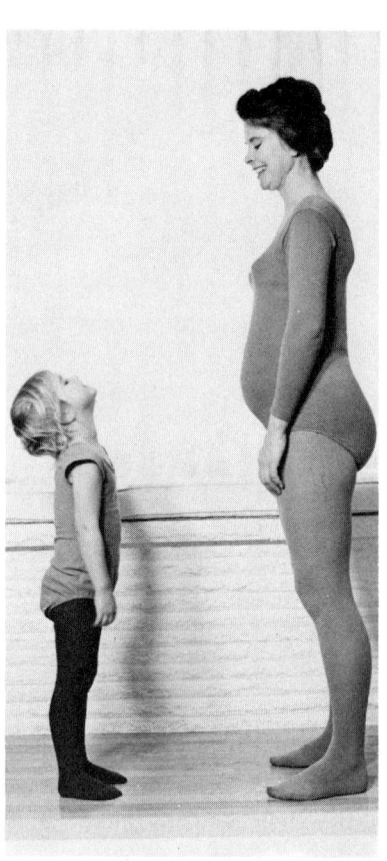

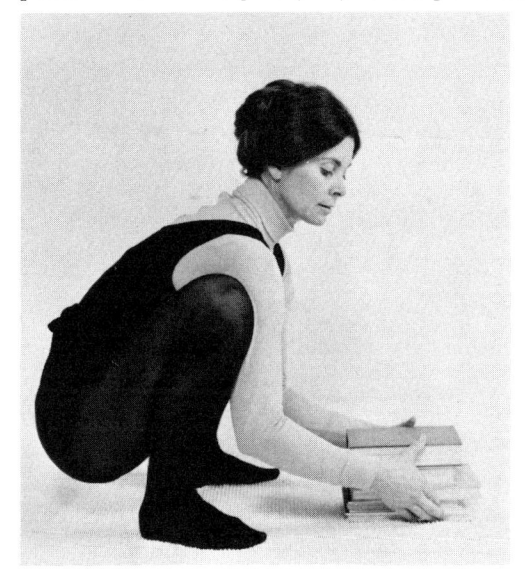

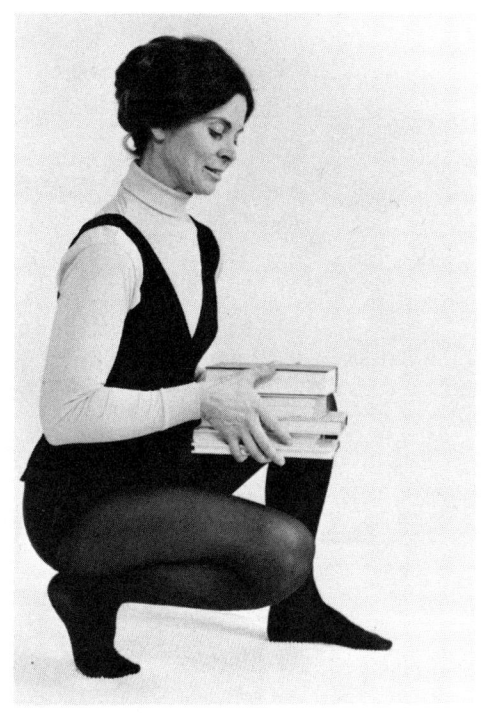

Lifting posture. When lifting anything heavier than an article of clothing from the floor, use your legs and *not* your back. Change your posture from the squat (left) to the position on the right. Now you have better balance because of a much larger base. Notice the area of floor if you draw an imaginary square around your feet; compare this area with that of an ordinary squat. Now you can use your leg muscles without fear of falling. Since pregnancy sometimes causes slight dizziness as you change position, a chair or table nearby can be grasped with one hand to steady you.

This is a lifetime habit for you to learn. When not pregnant, you can rise from the original squat position with your back straight, since you do not have a heavy uterus to overbalance you, but this way is much easier and more graceful.

Remember to lift with your legs, not your back. This is **also a** useful posture for reaching the baby in a crib or bassinet. Use your legs and keep your back straight.

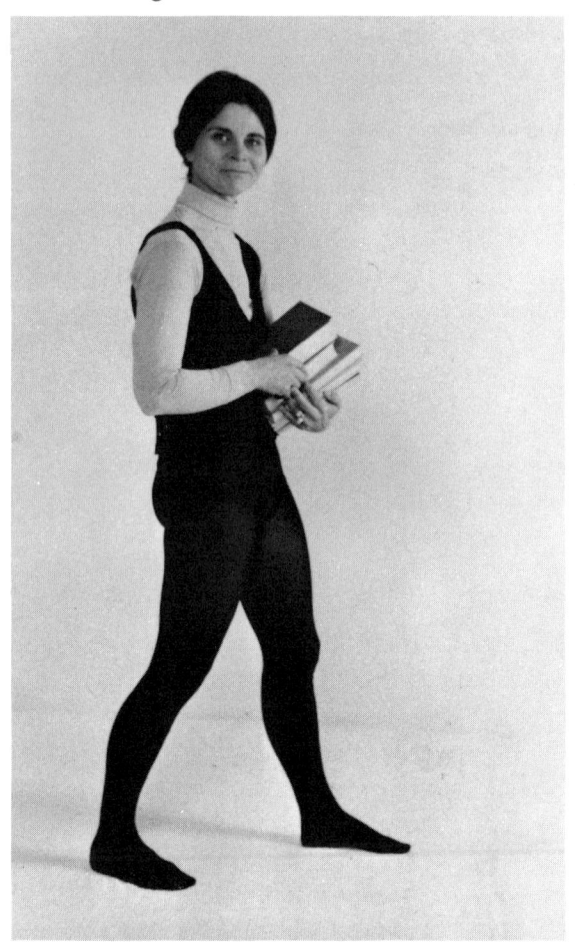

CLASS TWO

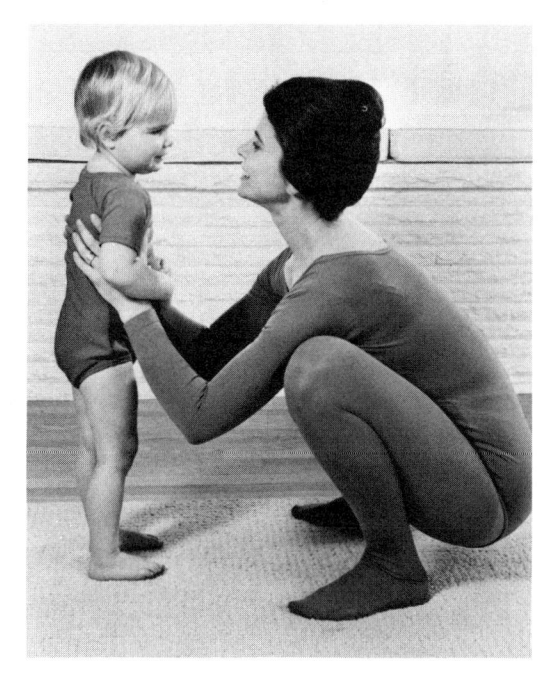

Leg Cramps
Heartburn
Eating for Two
Variations of Pelvic Rock
Sitting Pelvic Rock
Standing Pelvic Rock
Kitchen Sink Pelvic Rock
Butterfly

    The class personality has changed a great deal in one month's time. There is a definite assurance about everyone that was missing before. Of course, it helps to know how to get to the class, where to park, and who the instructor is—but it seems to be more than that. You are willing to be one with other class members despite your differences. Pregnancy is a bond stronger than other qualities. You've thought of lots of questions lately and are ready to talk about them.

    It seems that you've worked through most of those early new feelings about being pregnant. You are becoming comfortable with your new state of being. It's still exciting, but not so scary. Your tummy is still a bit small for regular maternity clothes, but you cannot wear all your nonpregnant things anymore. You've noticed changes in your body. Your breasts may be tender and enlarging. You may have darkened pigment on your face, tummy, and nipples. You may still have that awful nausea, but you've discovered that it is not going to get any better by thinking you are sick, so you are trying to ignore it. No one gives you any sympathy for it anymore either—especially your husband. He's as tired of it as you are.

Your baby is kicking now. Those movements in your abdomen that you thought were intestinal grumblings are probably the baby bumping around. He is still terribly small—about seven inches and four ounces—but is a complete being. That's a lot of development in four months.

The baby's birth seems so far off, yet you feel as though you've been pregnant forever! It's a good time to work harder on relaxation and abdominal breathing.

You've been getting many questions about natural childbirth from all directions. You are now really aware of how necessary it is to be able to explain what you are planning to do. Your husband, too, may be getting lots of comment, which may have either turned him into a fanatic or made him a little suspicious. The two of you may need to study up a bit on the subject. If you have not already read *Husband-Coached Childbirth* by Dr. Bradley, now is a good time for it.

There is a pleasant, friendly feeling among you and your classmates by now. You recognize a really common bond with each other, especially now that you know the whole world is not appreciative of natural childbirth. You are probably trying to talk everyone you know into having a baby "our" way, and it's fun to find that all the class is having the same problem. As a matter of fact, almost everything one of you says has the rest of the class nodding their heads in agreement. In one small month you've all gone from *unsure* to *oversure*.

Leg Cramps

A common complaint of pregnancy is leg cramps, particularly in the calf muscle. It is easily treated by pointing your heel as you stretch your leg out straight. In fact, the cramp can be avoided if, as soon as you feel the crampiness beginning, you pull your toes toward your face —that is, point your heel. If, however, you are asleep and by the time you've wakened the cramp or "charley horse" is well established, then I advise standing, full weight, on the offending leg. You can give yourself a muscle spasm by pointing your *toe,* so do avoid that.

If you have a great many leg cramps, tell your doctor. He may have you stop drinking milk and prescribe calcium tablets instead for a while. This seems to help. Or he may discover another cause.

Remember, point your heel, not your toe!

Heartburn

Since we are discussing problems, shall we mention heartburn? It can be a plague of pregnancy. It is generally avoided by proper diet, and yet there are times when your healthy dinner and your baby seem to be fighting for space—which is exactly what is happening. Heartburn is just what it says: a burning sensation at the level of the heart. It is indigestion which becomes lodged in one spot, and it can be very uncomfortable. The first way to try to get rid of heartburn is to get up and move around; do the dishes, tidy the kitchen. If you sit slumped over in a chair watching television, it is sure to get worse. If you are still bothered after moving around, then try this:

1. Put your hands on your ribs at your sides.
2. Open your mouth and take deep, heavy breaths which push your ribs and your hands apart.
3. Do this several times.

In this way you give your stomach a bit more space, allowing proper digestion to begin.

Do I need to tell you to eat small, frequent meals? A daily portion of yogurt (about one-quarter cup) seems to help prevent heartburn in many cases. Sometimes a mint or chewing gum is helpful. Often a few sips of milk will bring comfort. Please try to avoid baking soda and antacids. We do not cut out salt (sodium) completely, but neither do we prescribe two teaspoonfuls at a swallow. Also there is evidence that antacids prevent absorption of B vitamins through the intestine. B vitamins are the energy vitamins—need I say more?

If you will recognize your heartburn as a warning that your diet and eating habits need reevaluating, I'm sure you'll solve the problem.

I am addicted to fiery hot Mexican food. Every once in a while I crave it. I like it so hot that my lips, throat, and tongue burn and tingle. You can imagine how my addiction and my pregnancies got along together! About every three months I'd not be able to stand it any longer; I would have my feast and I would suffer all night long. I guess it was worth it. Usually you'll know, too, why you have indigestion. It's talking yourself into doing without that extra piece of dessert, or the second helping, or whatever spicy foods seem to be the cause of your heartburn, that is hard.

Your pregnant body won't let you cheat—not in bad posture or in bad eating. You hurt when you don't take care of yourself.

It is vital that you have good nutrition, as the size and health of your baby depend on what you eat each day. Bad eating habits could cause stillborn babies, low-birth-weight babies, infection-prone babies, and even, in extreme cases, brain-damaged babies. Your diet is important for you as well as the baby: to prevent anemia; to prevent toxemia of pregnancy (a disease of late pregnancy symptomized by coma, convulsions, liver failure, heart failure, and even death); to protect you from severe infections; and to protect you from "natural" abortions.*

Let's begin Class Two with a discussion of eating!

Eating for Two

You need to become really diet conscious now that you are pregnant. An interest in eating correctly is important to your health, your baby's health, your energy, figure, and general happiness. Your primary concern is protein. That's the stuff of which bodies are made, and you are making a new body in your uterus. If you will eat a well-balanced diet and lower your carbohydrate intake, you will look and feel better. Most doctors like to make individual decisions on how much weight you should gain. Dr. Thomas Brewer lectures his clinic patients in Richmond, California, that their weight gain does not matter but their well-balanced nutrition does. He does not restrict salt or any food but stresses a high-protein diet. You must listen to your doctor on nutrition, but none will argue with the need for extra protein.

I love nutrition—it's fun. But I'm no expert. How can I talk to pregnant women, though, without telling you what to put into your mouths? Probably the most controversial nutritionist of our day was Adelle Davis—and I love her ideas. In my opinion, she did more to make the average person aware of what he eats than all the other dietitians in the country. She had a very practical approach to nutrition and tended to tongue-in-cheek comments. Her sense of humor is very obvious in her writing. Her most vehement critics often have never read her books! I find that cooking from her cookbook is an adventure. Baking potatoes

* Thomas H. Brewer, M.D., *Metabolic Toxemia of Late Pregnancy. A Disease of Malnutrition* (Springfield, Ill.: Charles C. Thomas, Publisher, 1966).

turns into a whole new production. Boiling beets is new and different. I enjoy knowing why white flour makes a different dough than whole wheat. So I suggest you try reading her books to see if she makes you as excited about nutrition as she does me. Beware of reading one chapter and going on a "one-vitamin binge." Read the whole thing, and do not take small bits of information out of context. Use her ideas on good, well-balanced eating and try to avoid curing your next-door neighbor's asthma. Adelle Davis was the expert—not you and I!

You may have to change your eating habits completely to become a well-nourished, healthy person, and now is a good time, while you are so conscious of your body. You do not have to eat three meals a day. Six may be much better for you. Throw out all the old ideas and start fresh!

The best protein comes from animal sources—meat, fish, eggs, cheese, and milk. Vegetable proteins do not have all the essential amino acids and cannot be used properly in your body as builders unless you supply the missing amino acids. So when you use vegetables for your source of protein, you need to put the correct combinations together. Beans and Boston brown bread give you complete protein. Peanut butter must be eaten with milk to make its protein available for use. Always use nonhydrogenated peanut butter or the protein is not available at all (you may have to get it in a health-food store or make your own!). Many of the typical native dishes have been put together with this good common sense. Mexican natives eat beans and corn tortillas. The native Italian peasant uses pasta, cheese, and a dark wheat bread. The Chinese use a large variety of vegetables (most vegetables have a small amount of protein) and soy beans. Soy beans are the best single source of vegetable protein.

Eating well can be a challenge, and much fun can be had in planning and preparing food. Here is a very general guide to a well-balanced daily diet during pregnancy:*

Meat, fish, beans, or cheese	Two servings.
Eggs	Two a day. This may conflict with some advice you will get, but egg is probably the most perfect protein you can eat and is a very good source of iron.
Milk	One quart a day (four glasses). The cheapest, easiest source of good protein

* Adapted from *Metabolic Toxemia of Late Pregnancy*.

	and calcium, which is necessary for the baby's bone development and nerve cells.
Vegetables	At least one green leafy vegetable each day and a yellow or red vegetable each day.
Fruit	At least one citrus fruit each day—orange, grapefruit, or lemon—plus other fruits.
Cereals and bread	One serving each a day of whole-grain cereal and bread made from whole-grain flour (two slices).

Vegetables and fruits provide a wide assortment of vitamins and minerals for general health, and the more variety, the better. Fruits and vegetables are also the best source of carbohydrate in a well-balanced diet. They provide nature's unrefined sugars and starches, whereas white sugar, candy, and soft drinks are carbohydrates with no vitamins or minerals—only calories. If you eat well, you will not have a craving for such empty calories.

Bread and cereals do not mean cakes, cookies, doughnuts, and prepared refined breakfast foods. Generally, whole-grain, less refined foods will taste better, satisfy you more, give you more nutrients, and keep the calories down.

Skim milk is as good a food as whole milk except that it lacks vitamin A, which is in the butter fat, or cream. You can afford to lose the butter fat but the vitamin A you must get in other ways (vitamin A enriched margarine, canned pumpkin, and apricots are some very good sources).

It is important that you gain enough weight to have a happy pregnancy and a healthy baby, but you do not have to change your own size by too many pounds. It's very hard to gain fifty or sixty pounds by eating sensibly and properly—it's possible, but not likely. Yet it's better to gain weight than to eat a poor diet. Usually the pounds go on with pie, cake, cookies, doughnuts, candy, and whipped toppings—none of which are important health-giving foods. Rarely do fruits, vegetables, enriched breads, eggs, fish, meat, and milk create a fat person—you get too full to eat too much! The food is satisfying enough to keep you from overeating.

Some oil is necessary in your diet for the absorption of vitamins A and D. This does not mean that you should eat fatty meat, oily gravies, and butter-laden bread. A tablespoon of vegetable oil used on a salad would be sufficient for your needs.

A meal that looks pretty is very often rather well balanced. If you have different colors and shapes and consistencies of foods, you will usually be balancing the nutrients. Likewise, a variety from meal to meal and from day to day will help balance the nutritional content. Try to eat a different kind of meat each day during the week. Use meat substitutes for some meals—beans and cheese or fish. Try a different salad with each dinner. Prepare a new vegetable or one you seldom eat. Experiment with new greens—try tossing a salad with oil and vinegar and your own choice of spices. Concoct, create, try new things. Do not serve the same color, shape, or texture of vegetables at one time. Mostly, avoid serving the same old thing seven days a week! Day-to-day food planning can get very dull unless you make it fun. You will become invigorated and feel excited about meal preparation. You are challenged in these nine months, and on into the months you will breastfeed, to eat the most nutritious food you can for the sake of your baby. Make it an adventure. Let meal planning be one of your specialties.

If you eat foods that are natural—that is, as close to their original form as possible—you will probably get more food value and will spend less money on food. Buy whole potatoes rather than powdered mashed potatoes. Buy fresh vegetables rather than frozen and frozen rather than canned. Of course, home-grown vegetables are best, since they come directly from the garden to the table. If you've ever grown your own you know that even the taste is better. Whole-grain cereals are more health-giving than refined, sweetened dry cereals. Whole grains ground into flour are more nutritious than refined, bleached flours. Convenience foods are generally of low nutritional value and very high cost. I am generalizing, and that is dangerous; there are exceptions to everything. Powdered milk is cheap, and its nutritional value is just fine!

We are all creatures of habit, and many things we eat just because we've always eaten them. I ask you to begin thinking carefully about your diet and toss out those unimportant foods for quality ones. If your doughnut for coffee break and chocolate bar before bed are more important to you than ten extra pounds, that is your choice; but don't leave out your daily orange and your two servings of vegetables to subtract the calories furnished by the doughnut or the chocolate bar.

You are in for a great treat if you've never looked into the composition of foods until now. It is really exciting to see what foods contain. It's sometimes surprising that what you feel guilty about eating is really good for you. I remember a friend eating only the crusts of bread and not eating the center of the slice because it was not as good for her! The fact is that B vitamins are destroyed by heat so the crust is not as rich in vitamin B as the center of the slice. (Of course, if you're eating white bread, you're not getting much out of it anyway.) Find out what it has in it that's good for you, and you can justify eating it—maybe!

Let me say a word to the vegetarians. I admire you. Of all the people I know, my vegetarian friends are the most conscious of good, well-balanced nutrition. It takes much knowledge of the composition of foods to be a healthy vegetarian. It is more difficult to get sufficient protein and iron when you do not use the easy source—meat. Since protein is so vital to you while pregnant, keep counting your grams and enjoy!

What I ask of each and every one of you is to become curious about what you eat. Look up the value of each thing you eat to find out whether it's good for you or not very important nutritionally. Become selective. Here is a time in your life when your eating habits directly affect another human being. Surely you care enough to provide the best possible chance of having a perfectly created baby. I'm not asking you to become a fanatic about one style of eating or another. You can have a healthy, well-balanced diet from the supermarket; from eating vegetarian foods; growing your own crops organically; taking vitamin pills as supplements; eating wheat germ, liver, and brewer's yeast till you get to like them; or having to stick to a medical diet. Do your own thing with food, but make sure you give your body adequate protein, carbohydrates, and fats, plus all forty vitamins, minerals, and essentials for good health. I have given you general ideas only. Please find a good reference on nutrition, and make sure you follow it. Write or phone the Department of Agriculture or your County Extension Agent and ask for nutrition guides. Especially valuable is "Nutritive Value of Foods," U.S. Department of Agriculture Home and Garden Bulletin No. 72. Another source of good diet information for pregnancy is Nutrition Action Group, Box 1346, Richmond, California 94802. Their pamphlet is entitled "Pregnant? and want a healthy child."

Variations of Pelvic Rock

By now you will be adept at all the postures and exercises you learned in Class One. Maintain them all, adding the new ones we present in Class Two.

Since pelvic rocking is so vital to your comfort and health during pregnancy, we have provided additional positions. The hands-and-knees position is by far the most effective means of "rocking your pelvis," so use it whenever possible, but these other methods will give variety to your pelvic rocking and can be used during the day as you do your routine activities. You will be able to rock your pelvis when sitting and standing, as at the kitchen sink. By maintaining a straight spine with the help of these postures, you will feel infinitely better all day long. You are also taking care of the uterus by tipping the pelvis forward, releasing pressure, and allowing good circulation. These variations count as your daytime pelvic rocking, but before bed only the hands-and-knees position is allowed.

You will become addicted to pelvic rocking. At least I have! Nothing makes my back feel so good. I still routinely do my pelvic rocking before bed and have discovered that I maintain a strong back, good posture, and tight tummy muscles as a result. I recommend that you, too, consider pelvic rocking a lifetime exercise.

If you are doing these variations in front of others, such as while you sit at your typewriter at the office, it may look a little less conspicuous if you do them one at a time, with rather long intervals in between. Sitting at your desk, violently working away at pelvic rocking, you may cause a minor riot at the office. Standing pelvic rocks in front of the filing cabinet will brand you as a belly dancer—at least. These "exercises" are nothing more than basic body movements and can be performed quietly and unobtrusively as a stretch or change of position. They *can* be used to get attention, though, if you want to teach about natural childbirth.

Sitting Pelvic Rock

Though the sitting position is not as effective as the other methods of pelvic rocking, the advantage is that it can be done while you are sitting doing routine tasks. It will relieve back tension and pelvic pressure.

HOW

1. Begin in a tailor sitting position. Roll your pelvis back so that your weight shifts to the base of your spine. You feel as though you have been pushed in the abdomen.

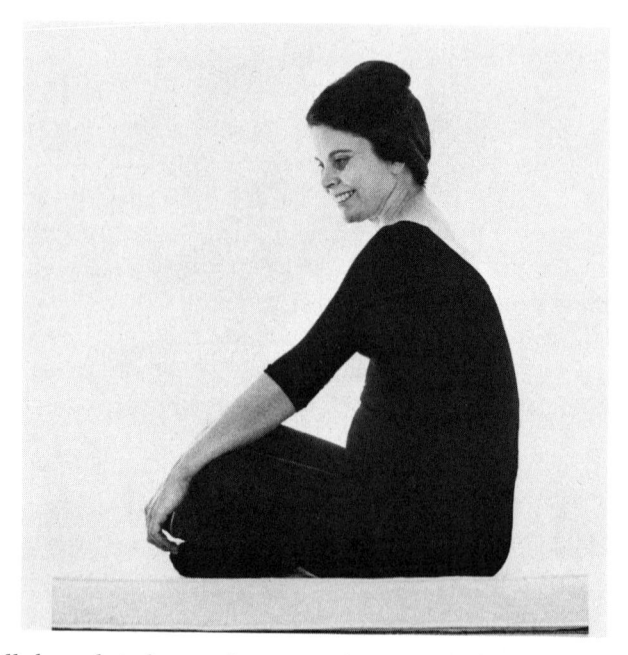

2. Roll the pelvis forward again as far as it will go.

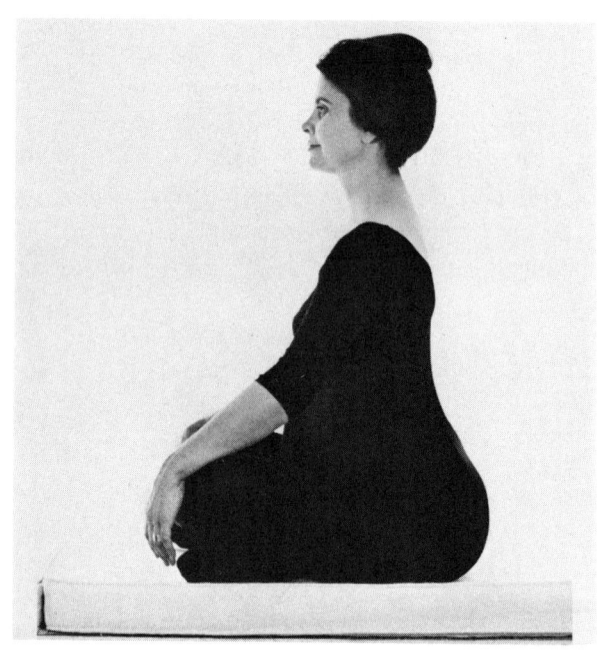

3. After repeating these motions about ten times, stop when the pelvis is forward but relaxed.

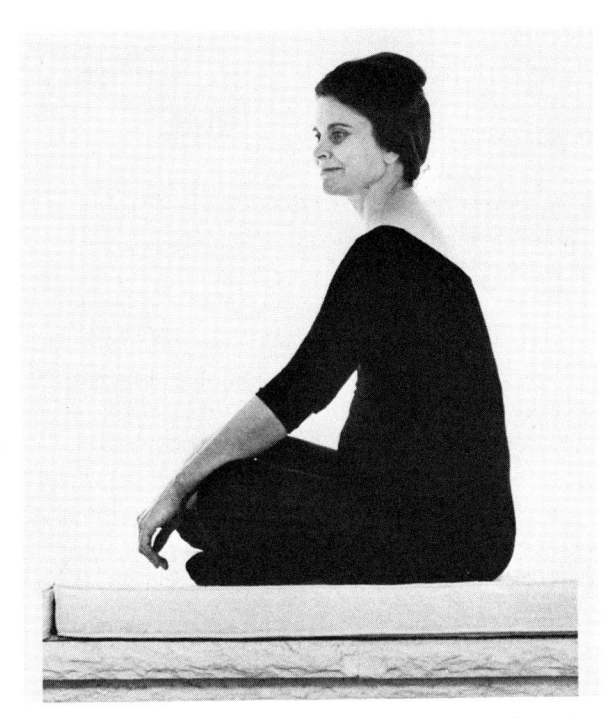

WHERE If you are not able to assume a proper tailor sit position on the floor, you can do the pelvic rock sitting in a chair. Try to get yourself out of the habit of crossing your legs when sitting in a chair. This contributes to poor circulation and may also help to build "saddlebags" on the sides of your thighs.

Pelvic rock sitting can be done: at a desk at the office; at a sewing machine; at the beauty shop (especially under the dryer); at the movies (it's especially easy to do at a drive-in, where you can tailor sit, but don't forget to use it in a theater, too); in a car (especially important during long periods of riding); while watching TV; reading; knitting. Whenever you are sitting, do occasional pelvic rocks.

WHEN Midmorning, noon, midafternoon, early evening, and anytime in between. They can be very unobtrusive if done one at a time.

Standing Pelvic Rock

This posture is extremely important since we all stand a great deal, despite our inclinations to the contrary! Standing pelvic rock should be learned so well that your posture will improve (unless you already *have* perfect posture). Pregnancy is a good time to better your postural habits, since you become uncomfortable so easily now, standing or sitting or lying with bad posture. So you have a built-in correction system —*do* use it.

Standing pelvic rock is especially good to build strength in the back muscles and to maintain a good posture while standing.

It makes you look better because it lifts your chin, raises your breasts, strengthens your shoulders, tightens your buttocks, pulls in your abdomen, and unlocks your knees. You appear to the world as a woman proud to be having a baby. You look and feel two months earlier in pregnancy than you would with a sway-back and a protruding abdomen. You do not outgrow your clothes as quickly; therefore, it is helpful to your clothes budget. You can button your coat and may not have to buy one especially for your pregnancy. (For those of us in cold climates, this is rather important.)

Standing pelvic rock gives a slight relaxation to the knees and thus aids leg circulation. Varicose vein troubles are lessened. Add to all this that it keeps you from walking like a duck!

If your back is kept straight it will not ache from the weight of the baby tugging on the muscles and ligaments that connect the uterus to your back.

Some of the stretch of the abdominal wall will be eliminated. One of our class members exemplified how very stretched the abdominal skin can become. She had had three pregnancies prior to taking our classes. Her figure was good, but she had allowed that heavy uterus to pull her abdomen forward. When she did the standing pelvic rock in class for the first time, her dress became tucked between her ribs and abdomen because she had so much stretched loose tissue and skin. She looked so much better and had no back tension after learning this simple posture tip.

The amount of loose skin on your abdomen after the baby is born will depend a great deal on how well you have maintained a good posture throughout your pregnancy. The baby doesn't ruin your figure—you do! If you will use plenty of lubrication on the skin (any kind of skin oil that you like to use) and hold your uterus in your pelvis while standing (keeping buttocks tight), you will have as pretty a figure for a bikini as you ever had—after the baby, that is!

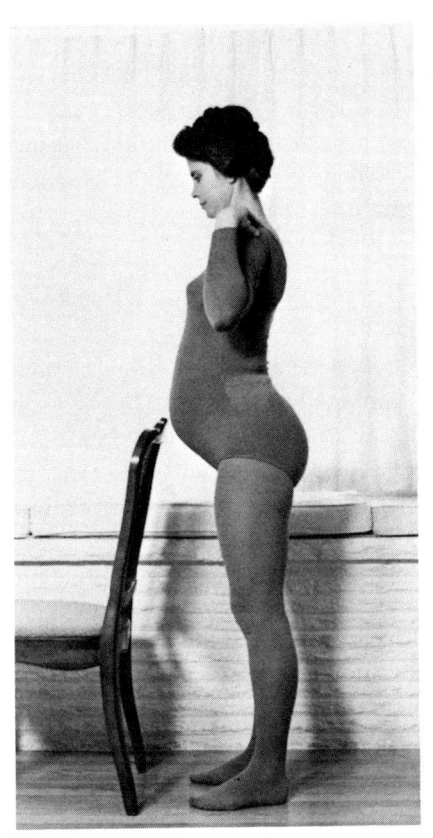

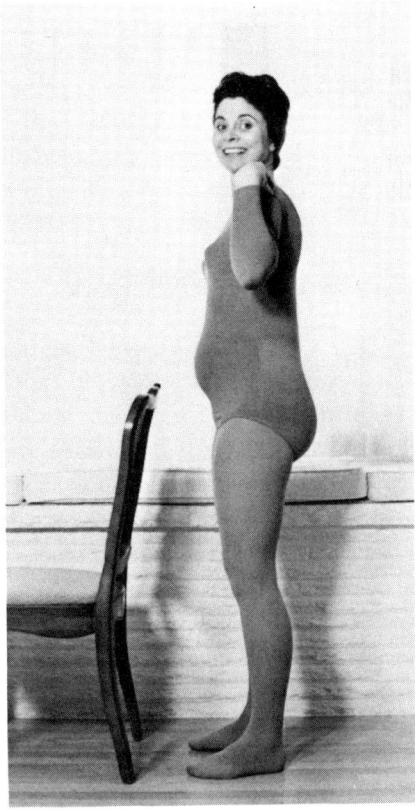

HOW

1. Put your hands on your hips so that you can feel the pelvic bones. (I've kept my hands up so that you can see the posture more clearly.)
2. Push your hips and abdomen forward and tailbone back and up (toward the ceiling).
3. Reverse. Tuck your tailbone under you and tighten your buttocks. The top of the pelvis has moved back, bringing the hipbones with them. Notice how your abdominal wall has tightened.
4. Repeat 2 and 3.

WHERE AND WHEN Standing pelvic rock can be done anytime you are standing, such as: waiting in line at the supermarket; waiting to cross the street; when you get out of bed (it will help you get moving in the morning!); every time you look in a mirror; when you get out of a car; getting up after sitting on a sofa; every time you feel tension in your back. Obviously, this movement can be done any time you want to, or remember to do it! It can become such a habit that you'll do it all day long. Eventually your spine will become permanently straight because the muscles are strong and developed. When you are no longer pregnant you should continue to do this to maintain good posture.

Kitchen Sink Pelvic Rock

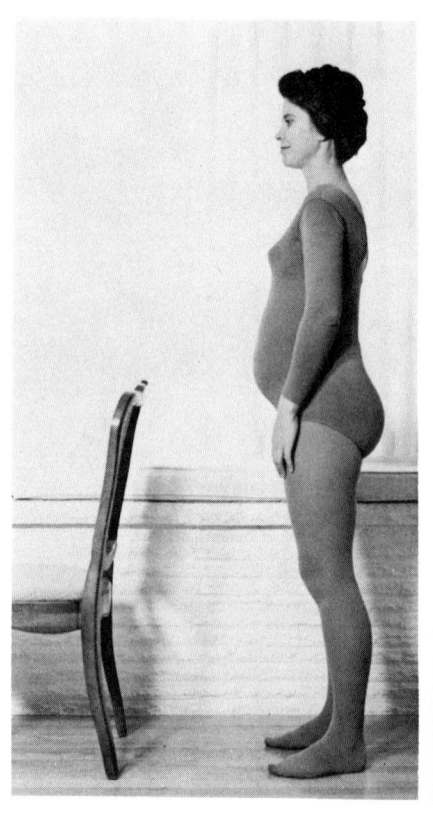

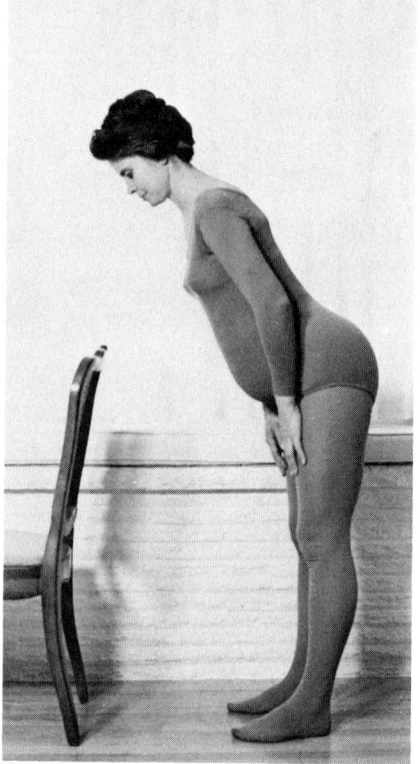

This exercise was taught to me, personally, by Mabel Lumm Fitzhugh. She was a dear, vivacious, limber lady who was probably in her sixties when I met her. She spent several days with us when I was being trained as a new teacher. She was also helping reevaluate our program. This exercise was added to our pelvic rock variations at that time. Its special quality is that it can be easily fitted into a busy day. The "kitchen sink" can be anything of the right height—a chair back at the office, the desktop in the schoolroom, a window ledge, bathroom sink, countertop, cupboard, dresser, etc.—wherever you are. We suggest the kitchen sink because it is a spot where you will spend much time if you are a homemaker. The exercise should be done each time you go to the sink (or to the chair at your desk, etc.). Through frequent practice you will maintain good posture and give yourself quick relief from pelvic pressure, as well as improved circulation to the lower part of your body.

Mrs. Fitzhugh used this exercise as a test on pregnant women in a clinic where no other form of exercise was encouraged. The women showed a marked avoidance of varicose veins and much less back discomfort than a control group.

HOW

1. Stand straight about two feet away from the sink, with feet comfortably apart (about six inches). Distances will depend upon your size.
2. Bow to the sink!

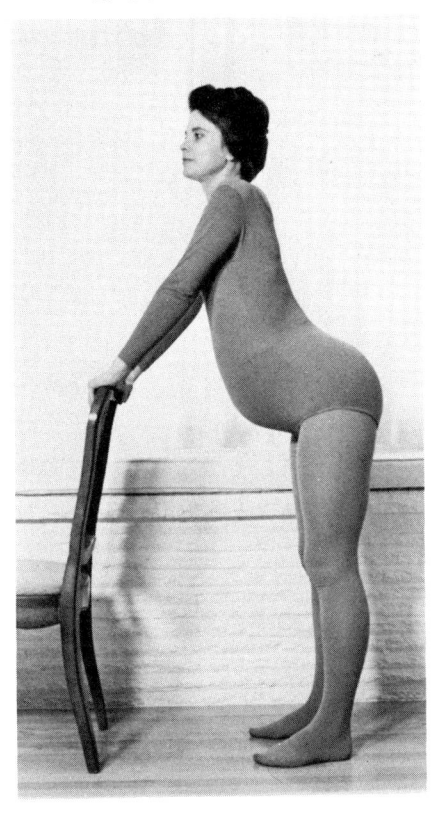

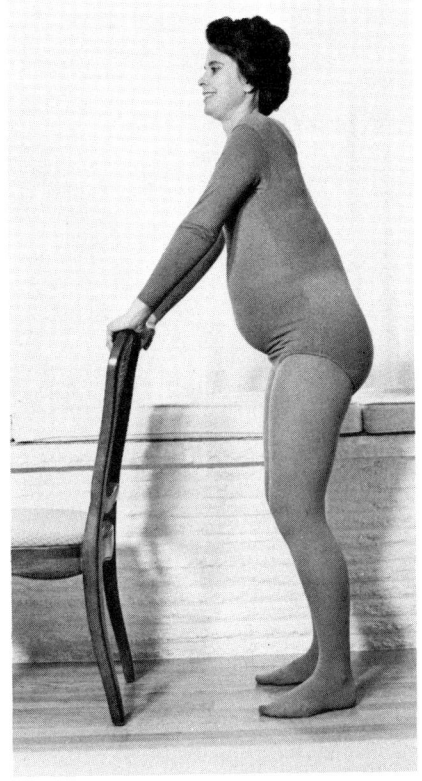

3. Put your hands on the edge of the counter, elbows stiff, and let your hands support your weight. In other words, lean against your hands.
4. Point your tailbone toward the ceiling. (It may hurt behind your knees, so go easy!)
5. Tuck your tailbone down and under you, as you relax your knees. This rolls your hipbones backward as your spine gets a comfortable stretch.
6. Do 4 and 5 three times.

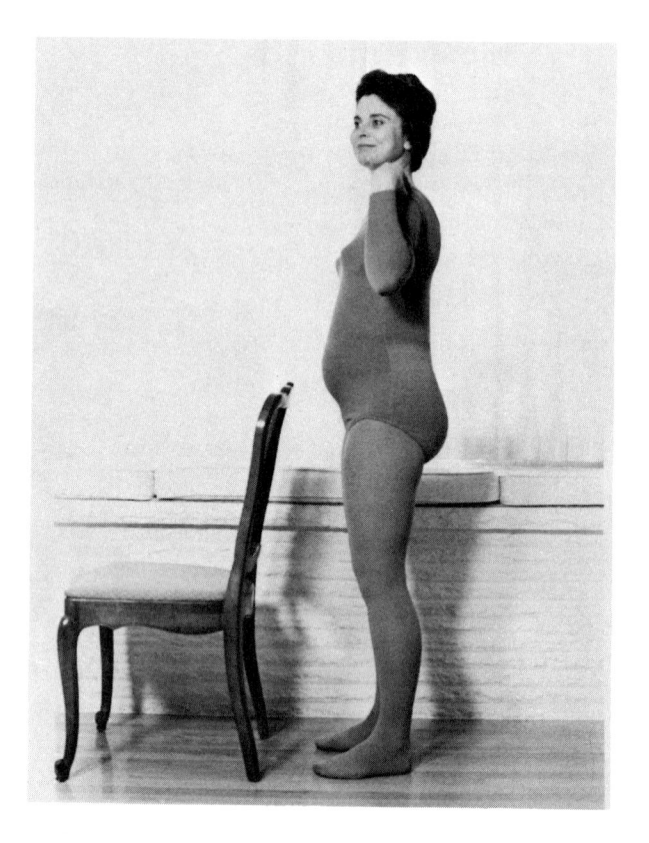

7. Now, with your lower back rounded, your tailbone tucked under you, knees relaxed, and buttocks tight, straighten your shoulders and head up over the rest of your body. Be sure to keep the good posture that you have created in the lower part of your back.
8. Walk up to the counter and find that you can get four inches

closer to it! Keep your knees relaxed and the same pelvic posture as you go on to other things.
9. Repeat each time you go to the sink!

WHERE This can be done at any table, counter, or desk that is the right height for you. If the counter is about the height of the top of your pelvic bone—about two inches below your waist—it is just right.

WHEN Do this exercise all day long, every time you go to your kitchen sink—or whatever chair or ledge you decide on as your point of most frequency during the day.

It may help you to remember if you write notes to yourself. When Debbie List, one of our teachers, was pregnant with Kelly, their son, she put a three-by-five card over her kitchen sink with "D.K.S.E." (Do Kitchen Sink Exercise) written on it. She used this idea effectively for other exercise reminders, too. Great idea!

Butterfly—or Legs Apart

This will strengthen the legs-apart muscles, or abductors.* Since they are weaker than the muscles that pull your legs together and since holding your legs apart is very important, especially during second-stage labor, the abductors need added strength.

Not only do you need your legs apart during a push, but between pushes, too, because the baby is low in the birth canal at this time. If your muscles have been completely fatigued with the effort to keep your legs apart during second stage, you may not have enough strength left to support you! Even if you don't walk immediately, you may have trembling, weak legs for several days if you have not prepared.

HOW Lie in contour position with knees drawn up and feet together on the floor.

Have your husband (our son Joe helped me with these photos) put his hands on the outside of each of your knees and exert gentle pressure as you push your knees apart as far as they will go. You may change your feet so that the soles are together—it's more comfortable.

Bring your knees back together (with no pressure against them) and repeat twice more, with slightly increased pressure each time you spread your knees apart (like a butterfly's wings).

* See *Husband-Coached Childbirth*, p. 112.

Warning about your husband: He is almost certain to have more strength in his arms than you do in your legs, so if he prevents you from moving, teach him the rules of this game!

Most men think that if three times is good, three hundred is better. Not so here. Stiff abductor muscles make every movement painful. Plead with him to do it only three times! Also, this muscle, overbuilt, is not pretty on the female leg.

Do not let him exert pressure on your knees as you return your legs to the upright, beginning position. This would strengthen the already much stronger adductors—nullifying what we're trying to accomplish.

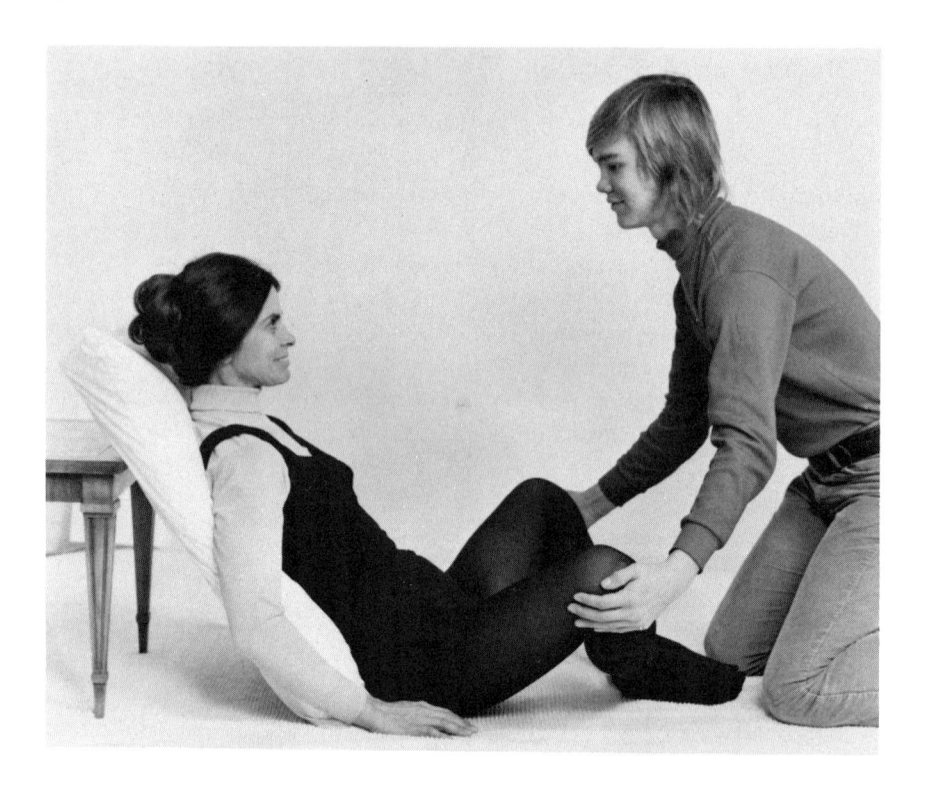

And do not let him push your knees to the floor as you are spread apart. Ouch!

You do not believe your husband will do any of these things to you, do you? Believe me, I have not made them up. They are experiences class members tell me about repeatedly—so I try to warn you in advance.

WHERE AND WHEN Wherever and whenever the two of you decide.

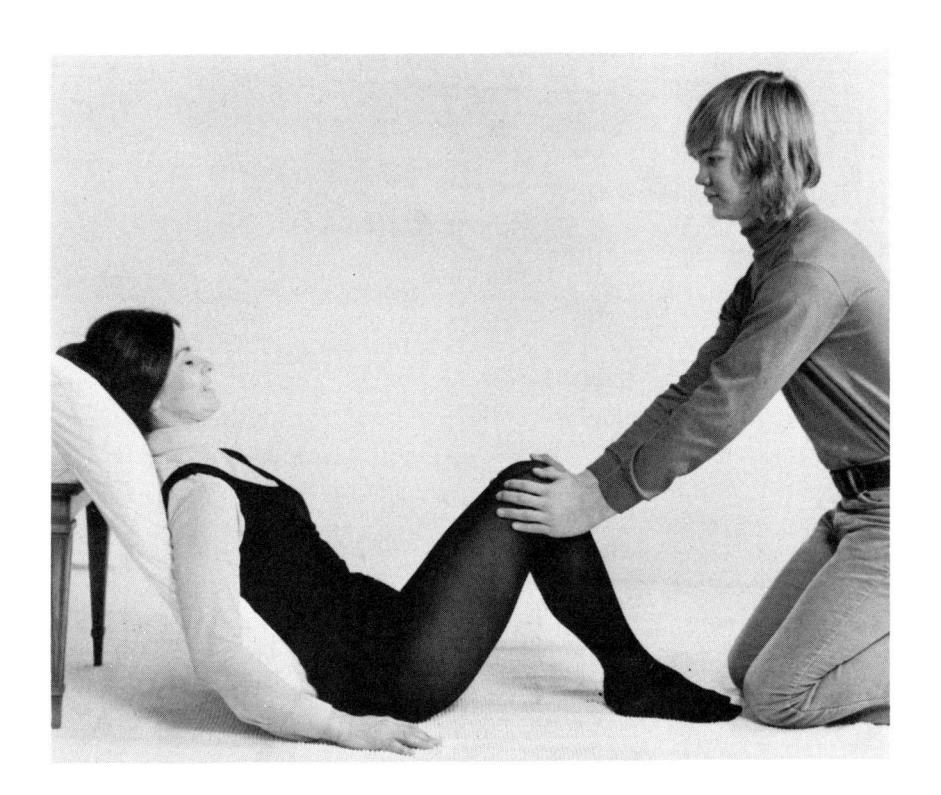

CLASS THREE

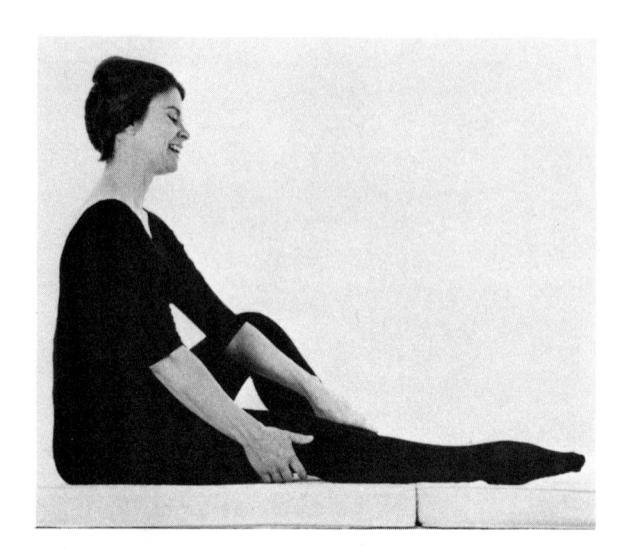

Kegel Exercise
Varicose Veins
Leg Elevation
Foot Circles
Leg Stretches
Breath Holding

You are in your fifth month and the baby is ten inches long and weighs about one pound. He has hair, his teeth have begun to form, and his bones can be x-rayed. The baby cannot live on its own yet, though.

You are now about halfway in your pregnancy and definitely showing. It's a time for comparing sizes with the other women in the class. There are great discrepancies between tummy sizes. Some of you look near term; others barely show. All inhibitions are lost among class members as they talk about their pregnancies. The fact that one is an intellectual working on her Ph.D. and the other is a ninth grade dropout —or that one has gobs of money and the other is on a subsistence income—or that one is a radical liberal and the other an archconservative —does not seem important as all contemplate being mothers. Pregnancy is a great leveler.

Confidence at this third class is very high. It's not uncommon for a class member to be assured enough to take over temporarily, relating her experiences or her point of view. Those who've had babies with us before are especially eager to tell the others "how it is." This is a help in teaching, as experiences shared with the class give good variety and bring up related matters that might never have surfaced otherwise. Questions are frequent at this class—even quiet girls become talkative.

Everyone has had two months to become proficient at the basic exercises. Tailor sitting is done easily and often. Abdominal breathing is by no means perfect, but usually comfortable. Relaxing needs more work but the idea is getting through. Pelvic rock is greeted with smiles and nods as we review it. Now we go into more new postures and movements which will help make your pregnancy more comfortable. It is time to begin practicing breath holding for the pushing stage of labor, so that will be included in this class also.

The middle trimester—or three months—is the most comfortable period of pregnancy. Your nausea is usually gone, or at least improved. The pregnant uterus is big enough to be riding up and out of the pelvis but not heavy enough to be causing too much pressure. Your mental outlook is generally superb.

So with this good attitude, let's learn some new postures for a healthier and happier pregnancy.

Kegel Exercise—
Tightening the Pubococcygeus Muscle

The pubococcygeus muscle is the floor of the pelvis, encompassing the perineal area. As its name indicates, it includes the area from the pubis, in front, to the coccyx, or tailbone, in back. It is the muscle that allows you to control the three openings all women have: the opening from the bladder (urethra), the opening from the bowel (rectum), and the vagina. Try to open or tighten each of these separately and you will find it impossible. They all work together because this one muscle controls the whole area. Learning to be conscious of the control of this muscle, and especially to maintain a constant tension in it, is our aim.

We call this the "Kegel muscle" and "Kegel exercise" after Dr. Arnold Kegel, emeritus professor of gynecology at the University of Southern California School of Medicine and director of the Kegel Clinic at Los Angeles County–USC Medical Clinic, who worked until his death in 1971 to help women understand their own functions.

Once I heard this handsome, white-haired, soft-spoken gentleman tell how he had begun his work some twenty to thirty years earlier by trying to prevent prolapse of the uterus in his gynecology patients. He taught them to squeeze the muscle that contracted the vaginal walls in an attempt to strengthen the support for the uterus. His patients responded as he'd hoped. After several months of exercising, they showed stronger muscular support in the perineum, which prevented further "falling" of the uterus. His patients began to disclose further benefits. Rather surreptitiously, they admitted that their sex life had improved. Dr. Kegel began to document the functions of the pubococcygeus muscle and started his lifelong crusade to help females understand how their bodies function and how to prevent physical inadequacy by a simple exercise.

Dr. Kegel's work and findings, as well as corroboration by other experts, are well documented in Ronald M. Deutsch's *The Key to Feminine Response in Marriage*.*

The role of this exercise and muscle is vital during pregnancy and postpartum. During pregnancy, the extra weight of the uterus stretches the pubococcygeus, which makes exercising it for strength very important. You know that a muscle which is used constantly is able to stretch and return to normal without injury and also is much stronger. A good healthy muscle, having good "tone," will be able to support a growing uterus for nine months and return to its usual function and size after the birth.

During the birth process, the Kegel muscle is put to a great test. It must have enough elasticity to move high into the vaginal wall and not impede the descent of the baby. You must be able to relax this muscle while pushing so you do not slow the birth. After delivery, the flexing of the Kegel muscle helps healing in general, and episiotomy healing in particular, if an episiotomy was necessary. The good condition of this muscle brings improved circulation to all the tissues in the area. Quick healing is promoted by good blood supply.

Stress incontinence during pregnancy is not uncommon—i.e., you may have a slight leakage of urine when you cough or sneeze. This problem should be effectively cured with "Kegeling."

For the rest of your life, the good condition of this muscle should be maintained. The proper alignment of your pelvic and abdominal organs depends ultimately on the Kegel muscle. An improper position, or a sagging or falling of the uterus, is called "prolapsed uterus," "fallen womb," or sometimes "tipped uterus." There are many names but it all begins with a uterus that is not exactly where it belongs. The symptoms are backache, heaviness in the pelvis, bladder infections, frequency of urination, incontinence (inability to control the emptying of the bladder), cystocele, and rectocele. Let me give an oversimplified explanation

* New York: Random House, 1968.

of cystocele and rectocele. As the uterus pushes downward into the pelvis, it pulls the adjacent tissues with it. This causes the tubes from the bladder (urethra) and the bowel (rectum) to get into abnormal positions. Pockets can form which make complete emptying of the bladder and bowel difficult. There is increased risk of infections as urine becomes "caught" in a pocket or cystocele. A pocket in the rectum (rectocele) causes alternate constipation (which may help develop hemorrhoids) and diarrhea as the blockage finally releases.

I have purposely listed these unpleasant "women's complaints" because the good tone of your Kegel muscle can help prevent them. Your sex life is another good measure of how well you've done your Kegels!

I admired Dr. Kegel and had been teaching this exercise and using his name for years before I finally had the opportunity to hear him speak.* I rushed up after his presentation to talk with him. I was very impressed by his soft humor and completely "proper" attitude to a subject that just begged for off-color remarks. He gave me his full attention in answering my questions. As he was explaining a point, he put his hand into his jacket pocket and pulled out a small white box. Opening it, he removed some cotton packing—as would be used with jewelry—and very gently pulled out the cast of a female vagina. I was speechless! He had developed a plastic which he could pour into a vagina, that would harden and set and could be removed within a few seconds. He then had an exact model and could show the "owner" her problems. If the pubococcygeus muscle was in good tone, with proper tension maintained, the vagina resembled a cylinder. If the lady was a mess, her vagina was more like a thick pancake. What a teacher he was! How could a lesson like that ever be forgotten?

HOW Tighten the "stopping the flow of urine" muscle. Now, as you tighten, pull up or lift with the tightening. "Tighten—lift—lift—let go." Count it so that with each tightening you lift to the count of three and relax to the count of two. (The whole count takes about two seconds.) This will help teach you the constant tension that should be present in this muscle. It should never be completely relaxed while you are awake.

The first time you try this, spread your legs apart, then tighten and release the muscle. Do not allow other muscles to get involved. Buttocks, thighs, and abdomen can be confused at first with the simple Kegel contraction.

* At the 1968 International Childbirth Education Association Convention, in Anaheim, Calif.

Since the Kegel muscle can control the flow of urine, start by trying to interrupt the flow of urine, while your legs are spread far apart. If you do this exercise five to ten times each time you void—that amounts to hourly exercise during a pregnancy! You will perhaps notice that you do not need to empty your bladder as often with a stronger muscle. You may not have to get up at 4 A.M. for a bathroom visit, but will be able to sleep until 6 A.M. instead.

WHERE Anywhere—any position. No one should be able to see you using this muscle as long as you are doing it correctly—unless you are like one gal in class who claimed that she could not do the Kegel without opening and closing her mouth, fishlike, at the same time. There really is no physical connection.

Talking on the phone is a good time to do twenty. You can brush your teeth and Kegel, watch TV and Kegel, stand in the supermarket line and Kegel, wait for a stoplight and Kegel, hold the door open for children and Kegel, dust the furniture and Kegel, pelvic rock and Kegel, stir the pudding and Kegel.

WHEN Twenty times each waking hour for the rest of your life. In other words, only when you are asleep should your Kegel muscle relax.

Varicose Veins

Do you understand what varicose veins are? It is a subject we should discuss, since the occurrence of "varix formations," as they are medically known, is higher in women than in men, and since the incidence in women increases with pregnancy.

Obvious varicose veins are ugly, tortuous, swollen blue veins that show on your legs—especially behind the knees. Sometimes there is nothing apparent on the legs because it is the deep veins that are varicosed. The degree of obviousness has no correlation with the symptoms produced. Some legs with obvious varicosities will cause no symptoms and another person who shows no varicose veins will have severe discomfort. Symptoms commonly are aching, tense legs with an itching or burning sensation of the skin, often accompanied by cramping of the calf muscle.

Varicose veins are aggravated by pregnancy for two reasons. First, the blood volume increases during pregnancy, causing an added burden to the circulatory system. Secondly, the main vessels of circulation to the legs run inside the pelvis, where the enlarging uterus is creating pressure. Since the pelvis is a bony structure, it causes a constriction of those arteries and veins. Our main concern is the inferior vena cava, which supplies the uterus. Arterial blood has the advantage of working with gravity but venous blood must fight an uphill battle. Further, the veins are not nearly as muscular and elastic as arteries (evolution made a small error there!). The veins do have valves which help prevent the backward flow of blood and the muscle tension of the legs helps keep blood moving, but that extra slowdown, as the veins are slightly compressed by the pressure of the uterus in the pelvis, can be the final straw. There begins a build-up of blood in the veins of the legs and instead of a fast-running river of blood, you have some "lakes" here and there. This destroys the elasticity of the walls of the veins and damages the valve system, so that backflow of the blood occurs, making the progress of venous flow toward the heart even more arduous. Stagnation of blood follows. The danger of infection in a vein (phlebitis) must be watched for, and ulceration of skin can also occur.

Is this enough to convince you that prevention is vitally important? Heredity is an added contributing factor to this whole picture. If your mother and/or father has varicose veins, your chances of the same are very high. But prevention and comfort are still important.

It should be mentioned, too, that anything wrapped tightly around your legs will inhibit the proper flow of blood, and could be a factor in causing varicose veins. Round garters and tight panty girdles should be avoided.

Support hose and elastic stockings, on the other hand, may bring comfort and relief to you who already suffer from painful legs. Your doctor can order special elastic stockings made to measure for you. You'll be much more comfortable, but you can help maintain good circulation with the postures and exercises that we'll explain in this class.

Remember that pregnancy does aggravate the condition, so that after the baby is born you will have less trouble or no trouble, depending upon the heredity of your veins. Work hard at these circulation exercises even though you have no apparent signs of varices. Small breaks in the capillaries of the skin are not varicose veins but are an indication of some distress and a good warning to you.

The following exercises are devised with circulation of the lower extremities in mind. Use them faithfully and you may virtually defy heredity, as I have done (at least so far). Leg elevation is really a treat so be sure to get the proper equipment ready and keep it handy. One good way to elevate your lower body is by raising the foot of your bed with three or four bricks. Your husband may not like the idea at first, but after a few days he may find that he is more rested and has lost that "woody" feeling in his legs. Men can have the same problem, even without a uterus!

Foot circles and leg stretches are easy, fast, and will get your sluggish circulation speeded up. Leg elevation will be helpful. Don't forget that hands-and-knees pelvic rock is one of the most important ways of eliminating pelvic pressure on those veins and getting the blood pushed through your circulatory system. I warned you that it would be a cure-all. "When in doubt, do some pelvic rocks" is our motto.

Leg Elevation

Varicose veins are a constant threat during pregnancy. Even though the problem lessens after the birth, the probability of some vein damage stays with you. So the more you can do to prevent any vein damage during pregnancy, the better off you are for life. Sometimes varicose veins will occur in the perineum, especially in the vaginal area. A symptom of this condition is pain and pressure in the perineum immediately upon getting out of bed in the morning. It is caused by the rush of blood to the area. You should find pelvic rocks on hands and knees helpful at this time, though leg elevation is the best relief and prevention position. Do lots of leg elevations to try to prevent any more damage to the veins. Lying on your back can be harmful, as it allows the heavy uterus to put undue pressure on the blood vessels (inferior vena cava), which results in oxygen deprivation to the uterus and thus to the baby. The kidneys, too, may be deprived of proper blood supply. Therefore, do your leg elevation for short periods of time only! Ten minutes is maximum. Although you are lying on your back, in what amounts to an inverted contour position, the reverse tilt of your pelvis virtually eliminates pressure. It feels so good that you may have to watch the clock to avoid staying in the posture too long. The gentle upward slope of the lower part of your body helps gravity return your blood efficiently to the heart.

HOW The idea is simple. You tip your head down and your legs up to allow the blood in the lower half of your body to flow back toward the heart.

The equipment can be simple, too. An inclined plane and two pillows. If you own a slant board, you have what you need. Tilt the bottom of it up about twelve inches, put a pillow under your knees, and you are set.

A contour chair or folding beach chair will do. Put your legs up the backrest and your head down. You may need a pillow under your lower back to be comfortable, and be sure that the backs of the knees are supported comfortably with a pillow. If too much contortion is required, don't use it!

An ordinary kitchen chair, with rungs, can be used with extra pillows, old blankets, or some good padding, as I have in the picture below.

You can make a slant board with a piece of wood as long and as wide as you are. You may be able to find a good piece of plywood in your husband's workshop—or go to the lumberyard. Wrap a blanket around the board and tie it on so that it won't slip—or upholster it with foam rubber, a pretty fabric, and upholstery tacks. The whole thing can be done rather inexpensively and you will not have to search for the makings every time you do the elevation. Prop up one end of the board on several bricks or the second step of your stairway, put a pillow under your knees, and you will feel fantastic.

In a pinch, an ironing board or large breadboard could probably be made into a workable solution. If you use a breadboard or a piece of plywood as I've used the chair in the picture, you'll need extra pillows to elevate your hips.

If your legs and feet begin to "fall asleep," be sure to slide off the slant board onto the floor or bed, assuming a side-lying relaxation position. If you do some hands-and-knees pelvic rocks next, it's a good time for a nap—but not on your back. When you get up, be sure to do it slowly to avoid the dizziness that often follows sudden rising from a prone position in pregnancy.

Leg elevation position.

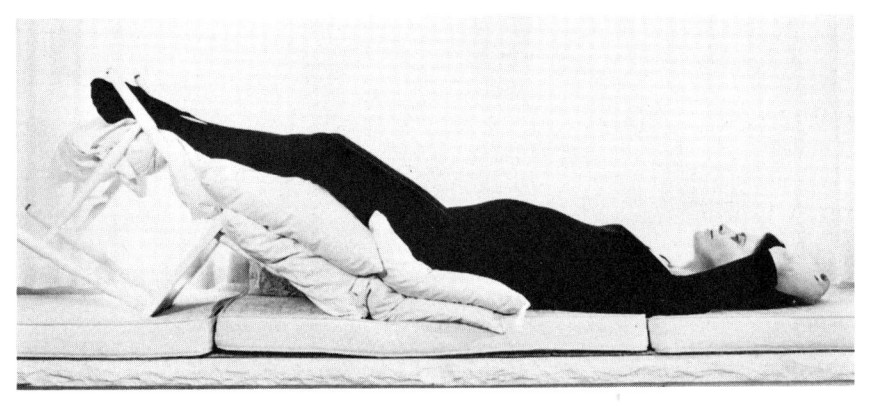

- Your head is lower than your heels.
- Your hips are elevated above your heart so that you can feel the uterus pulled up and out of the pelvis.
- Your knees are supported on a pillow in a slightly flexed, relaxed position.
- As the blood drains to the upper part of your body (which is now lowered), you may feel hot and flushed for a bit and your breathing may be "puffy."

Leg elevation exercise. To aid in circulation:

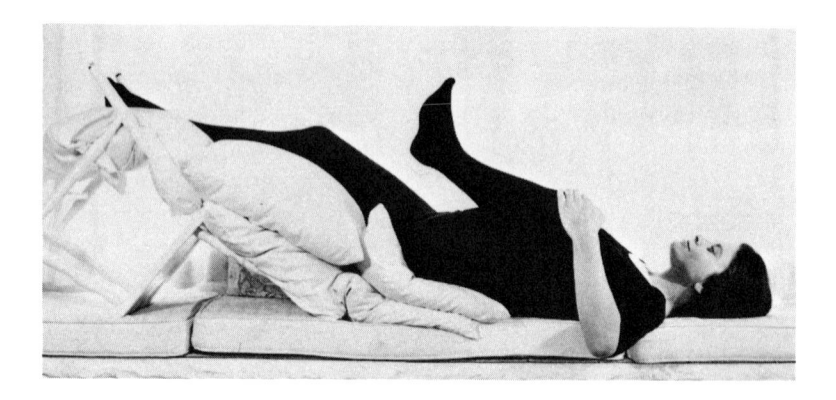

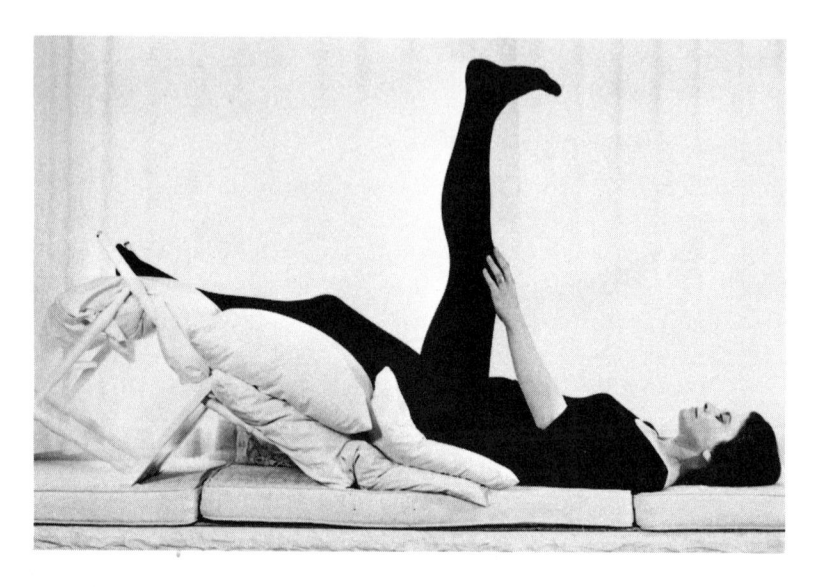

1. Bend one knee up toward your chest.
2. Straighten that leg up in the air with your heel pointed. (Do not point your toe or you may get a leg cramp.)
3. Lower the leg slowly to its original position, keeping your heel pointed.
4. Relax your leg completely and be sure the knee is partially flexed and slightly turned out.
5. Repeat with other leg.

WHERE Anywhere that you can set up an incline—with your head lower than your heels, a pillow under your lower back, and another under your knees to loosen them. It should be a handy spot so you are encouraged to get into this position often. Have the phone nearby and ignore the doorbell. It's also a good time for reading to a child or to yourself. If you are a slave to books as I am, you'll do anything as an excuse to read!

WHEN If you have varicose veins already, you will want to do this posture very often. Sometimes our doctors recommend that you put your feet up ten minutes out of each hour. Since you will be on your back, ten minutes an hour would be the *maximum* amount of time to spend in this position and anything up to that is O.K.

Foot Circles

This is another good exercise to help minimize varicose veins and it makes you feel better and more energetic, too.

By forcing the circulation of blood through your legs, you create an efficient exchange of nutrients and wastes to and from the tissues. It is better than a walk because the uterus does not become hammered into the pelvis to create pressure, as happens with walking. The good effects of walking when pregnant are nullified by the pressure created in the pelvis. So we do foot circles instead!

HOW

1. Lie in contour position with your left knee raised.
2. Rest your right ankle on your left knee.
3. Do a series of nine circles to the outside of your foot (clockwise).

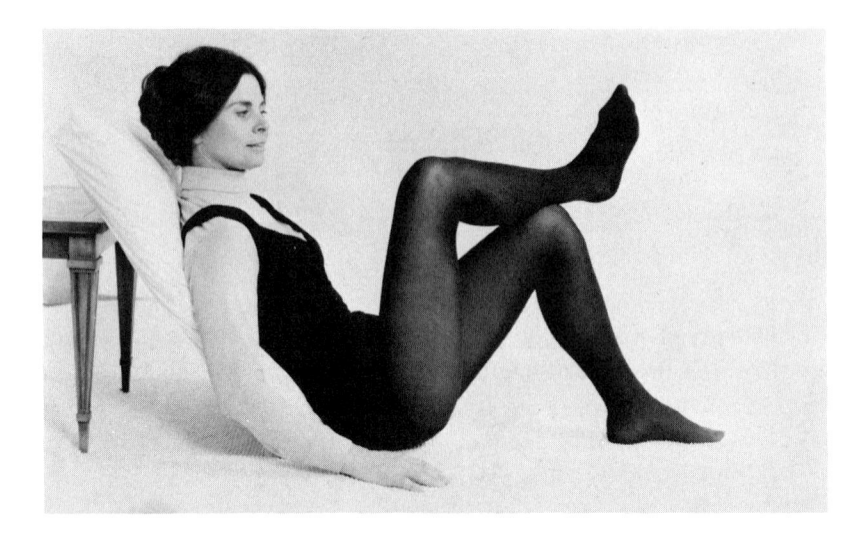

4. When you've finished nine circles, your toes are pointing up. Then relax your foot and shake out your whole leg, so that any muscle crampiness is released.
5. Do the same thing with the left ankle resting on the right knee, making counterclockwise circles.
6. Now enjoy the good feeling in your legs.

Think of tracing the face of a clock with your big toe. Start with your big toe pointing straight up to an imaginary twelve o'clock. Then your toes point to three o'clock, six o'clock, nine o'clock, and then twelve o'clock again. Do three quarter circles, three half circles, three whole circles, all clockwise. Do the opposite with the left foot—go counterclockwise. This will help strengthen the arch in your foot so that you need not be flat-footed with pregnancy.

WHERE Anywhere that you can relax and get into a contour position you can do foot circles. It's very comfortable to lean against your husband.

WHEN Do this anytime your legs feel tired. It is especially indicated if you've not rested sufficiently during the day. We can't control every day the way we'd like, so sometimes we need a revitalizing exercise and this one does just that for me. It is particularly useful when you have been shopping most of the day and have not done enough pelvic rocks (except the standing type while you waited for a clerk). You arrive home tired and the children are trying to punish you because you have been gone all day. Before dinner is begun, your husband arrives home. Perfect time for foot circles! Get the children involved in kiddie hour on TV or send them out to the sandbox, put a drink in the hands of your man (martini or apple juice) while you do foot circles and visit with him for a few minutes. You could do some hands-and-knees pelvic rocks, too, maybe take an extra five minutes and relax. Ask him to check your relaxation. Now you can go about your dinner preparations and the evening will proceed more smoothly because you feel better. You may not need to resort to tricks (that martini, the TV) to make time for your exercises, but do so if you must. Your pregnancy will be so much easier and more pleasant if you will take care of your body as the primary concern of the family.

It's easy to think, "I don't have time to do all these things," but what you are saying is, "I don't think it's important enough to take time." You are important and so is your baby in utero, which makes you *twice* as important.

Leg Stretches—
Flexing and Extending Ankles and Knees

Not only will leg stretches stimulate circulation in your legs; they will also strengthen your leg muscles and make it easier to carry those extra pounds caused by your growing baby. (You may even develop a more shapely leg!) You will be carrying your child for at least a year after he is born, too, so let's get ready now. If you wear high heels, this exercise will help stretch your Achilles tendon, which may have become shortened over the years. It is a good idea, pregnant or not, to vary the type of heel you wear (the lower the better).

Walking or running barefoot in sand is supposed to be the best exercise for your legs and feet. Sand moves under your feet as you walk to provide a workout for your muscles. Hard floors or cement sidewalks do not "move." One of our Denver teachers, Linda Scutt, claims to get this proper leg and foot movement from a specially built "Earth" shoe which is lower at the heel than at the instep. Since running barefoot in the sand is not possible for all of us, I've included these easy leg exercises.

HOW

1. From a tailor sit position, stretch one or both legs away from you at an angle, supporting yourself with your hands.
2. Point your toes away from you while stretching your leg out straight.
3. Pull your toes toward your body and raise your knee at the same time. The heel will rotate but for maximum effect it should not move from its position.

You can do legs separately or together until you feel comfortable. Resume your tailor sitting.

WHERE Leg stretches can be done anywhere you are tailor sitting—probably on the floor.

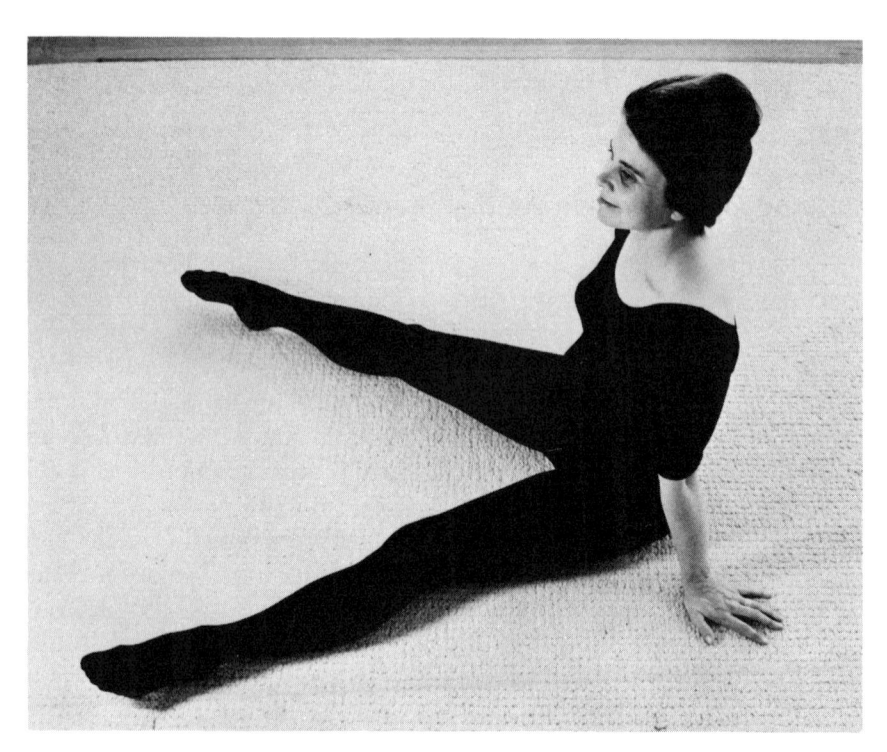

Extend: Toes pointed away from you, knee straight.

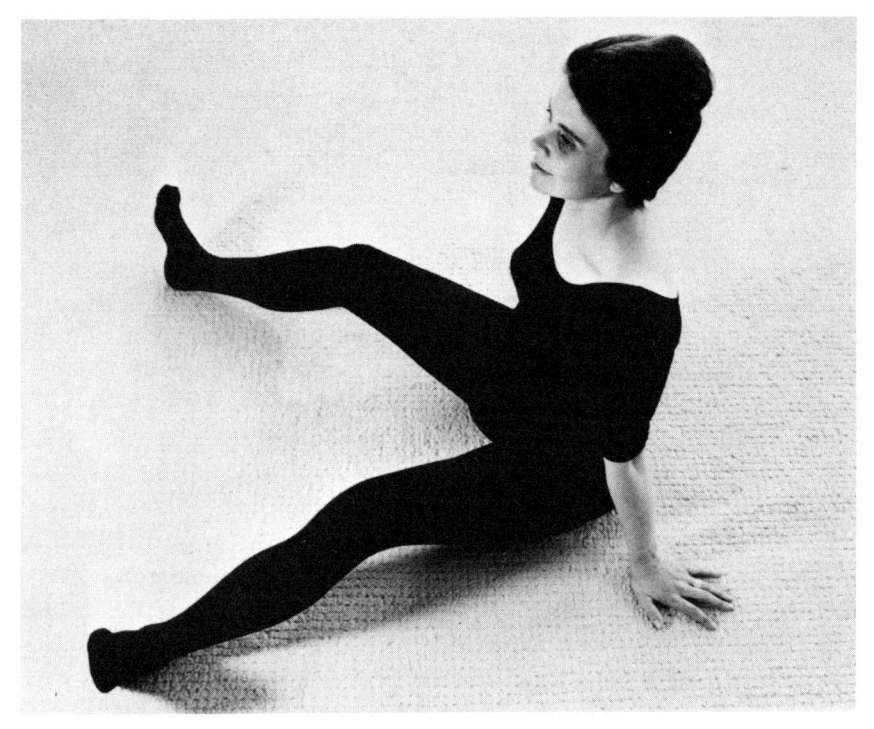

Flex: Toes toward you, knee up.

WHEN They are especially useful when you are involved in an activity and sitting in the tailor sit position. If you feel the need to move, but do not wish to interrupt your writing or reading—or simply do not have the energy to move around—this accomplishes the same thing.

Breath Holding— Breathing for Pushing

You are becoming proficient at abdominal breathing. Now let's learn the breathing for second-stage labor. First let me present my "nutshell" review of instructions for natural childbirth:

1. Use abdominal breathing and complete relaxation with each contraction in the first stage of labor.

2. Take complete, full breaths with each contraction in the second stage of labor and push as hard as you can while holding your breath.

It is important that you have a big breath to be able to push properly. Only with full lungs can you push down adequately with your diaphragm. The more usable oxygen you have in your lungs, the longer you can hold your breath and push. The longer you can push without having to replenish your breath, the sooner you will give birth! Each time you stop pushing to take a breath, the baby slips back in the birth canal. As you reapply the pressure of pushing, the baby descends and forces open the birth canal. Each push is a step forward; when you relax it's a small step back. This is truly hard work. Your body needs much oxygen and good, big breaths are necessary for effective pushing.

Learning to breathe properly for second stage will improve your efficiency.

The position for pushing is very important, too. In a squat position with chin on chest, all your energy is directed toward the baby, helping push the baby through the birth canal. It's as though your back is a bowstring pulled back as far as it will go. The baby is the arrow! The energy of the bowstring gives the impetus to the arrow. You will not be on your feet in a squat (though that would be ideal), but rather on your back, tilted into a forty-five-degree angle, with your legs pulled back and apart with your arms. You will be half sitting, with your husband supporting your shoulders. The other thing to remember—relax that baby door, the Kegel muscle. In this position, you can push your baby into the world efficiently.

HOW Tailor sitting posture seems best for practicing this breathing, but whatever position is comfortable for you is fine. The actual position that is used in labor—contour—may be uncomfortable during late pregnancy because the baby is so high up in the abdomen, making breathing very difficult as he pushes into your lungs. In second-stage labor, however, the baby has descended very low into the pelvis and in fact is at least partly in the birth canal, so there is plenty of space for the lungs to work properly.

To practice.

1. Sit comfortably.
2. Take a very large breath, until your lungs feel expanded. Exhale fully.

3. Repeat. (You have now taken two large breaths, exhaling each completely.)
4. Take another full, deep breath and hold.
5. Hold as long as you can—about forty seconds seems a good practice time. (As Dr. Bradley says, "No need for heroics!")
6. When you've held as long as you can, exhale fully.

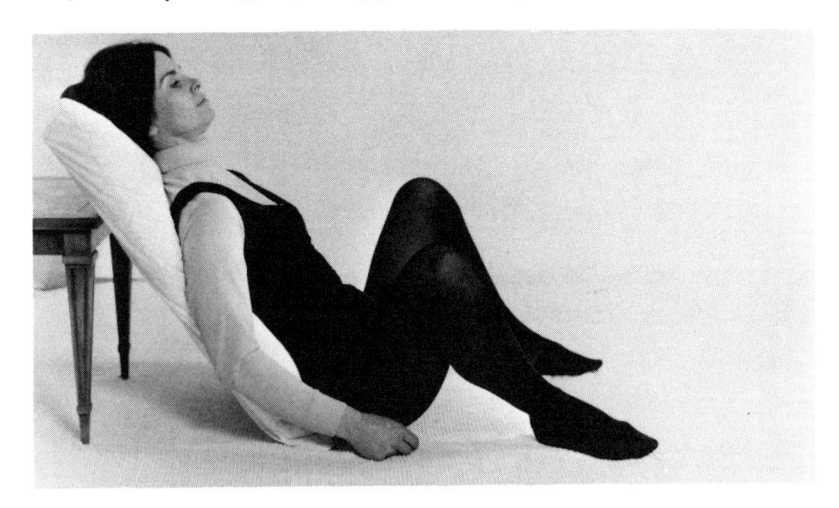

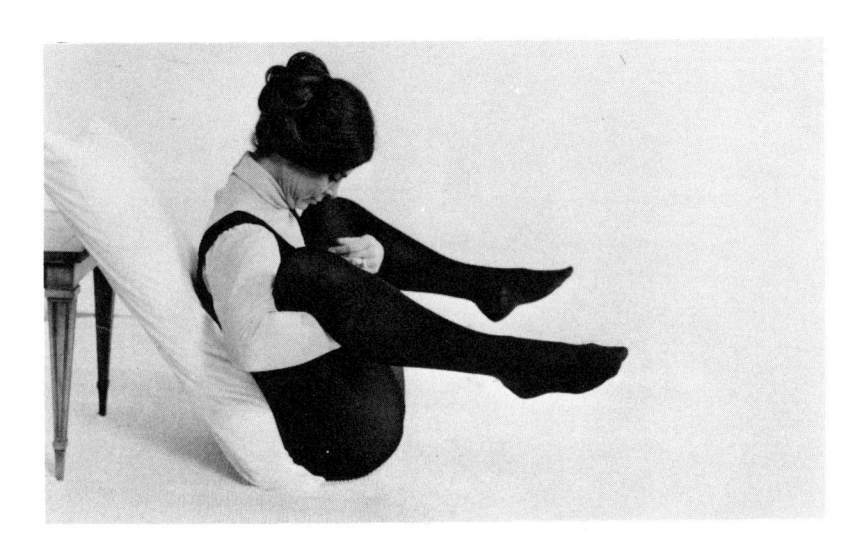

In labor. As you take your third breath, you will also be drawing your knees toward your shoulders and pushing them apart with your hands, and as you begin holding your breath you'll put your chin to your chest and bear down on the baby with strong, steady pushing. You will be nearly in a squat position, which is the most efficient position for giving birth. Keep your elbows out, pulling your knees apart rather than lifting your tailbone off the bed. You want to push the baby downhill, not uphill. When the pushing contraction is over, relax and wait for the next.

WHERE AND WHEN During labor you will use this breathing whenever and wherever you are when you receive that unmistakable urge to push!

Meanwhile, practice daily to improve your breath-holding ability. Have your husband rehearse with you since he'll undoubtedly hold his breath during your pushes in labor anyway. (It's automatic—have you ever tried to breathe normally while watching someone else hold his or her breath?) It will also give your husband experience in coaching for this final step of labor.

Practice the breath holding *only*. Practicing pushing will only contribute to hemorrhoids and is unnecessary, as those muscles are kept strong by your natural body functions, i.e., bowel elimination.

CLASS FOUR

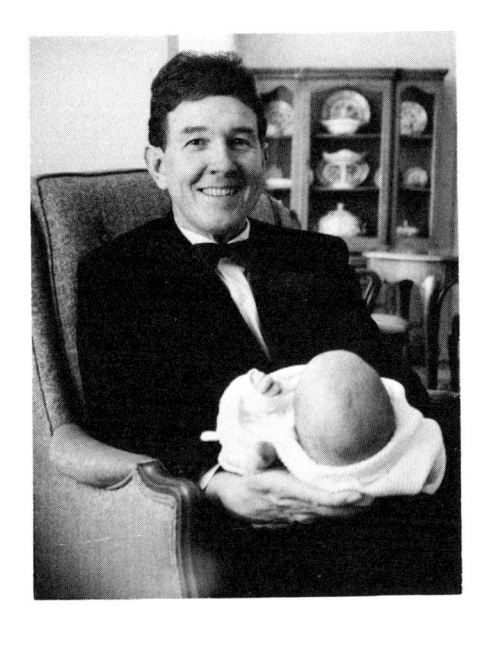

Breastfeeding
Bust Booster
Nipple Care

You are in your sixth month and your baby is fourteen inches long and weighs about two and one-half pounds. His eyes open and close and he has eyebrows and eyelashes. He has developed a layer of fat under his skin and is covered with vernix, a waxy, creamlike protective layer. Rarely would this baby live if born.

If ever you resemble the contented little mother image, it's probably now!

A new feeling is noted by this time. Six months have gone by rather speedily, all agree—but almost unanimously we wish we could hurry to full term. The weight of the baby sometimes becomes a burden now. It is getting to be more difficult to continue some activities. The trampoline artist must give up her show until after the baby is born! Bowling is a bit too challenging. The mother of three small children is feeling rather "worn out" by the end of a busy, chasing day. Many schoolteachers are required by the school boards to quit teaching at six months—which upsets most of them very much. Pregnancy in no way alters their ability to teach—run races, maybe, but not teach. This rule is gradually being changed.

You find lying on your back very uncomfortable, so even you confirmed back sleepers will manage to give up your habit with no trouble. It is absolutely not good for you to lie on your back. Those of you who tell me you wake up at night on your back are probably awakened by the discomfort. I doubt that you've been in the position long. If you are worried, have your husband check you in the middle of the night when you are asleep.

By Class Four you're ready for concentrated work on how to relax. Please review "Relaxation" in Class One. Be more critical of your performance. Try to improve. It's a good time to think about preparing yourself, mentally and physically, for breastfeeding, too.

Breastfeeding

We assume that anyone who is going to have natural childbirth is going to breastfeed her baby. The first nine months were natural; the second nine-month period should follow the same philosophy.

Breastfeeding is the most normal, natural, healthful, and satisfying method of feeding—not to mention the easiest and most economical! Once breastfeeding is established, it is the perfect supply-meets-demand system. The baby's need for milk automatically triggers the breast to produce the required amount. If the nutritional needs of the baby increase, he will nurse more often and/or suck longer and the breast will step up production of milk. It is a magnificent system, but of course, being human, we can throw it out of order. The insecurity of being one of the few people you know who have ever nursed a baby can be enough to put problems in your way. Many of you have never known anyone who nursed a baby. You thought breastfeeding was something that "primitives" do. Or perhaps the only woman you ever knew who did nurse her baby was someone you did not like. Does your husband want you to nurse his baby? These and countless other factors may influence your decision to breastfeed and your ease in doing so.

First you must understand the facts about breastfeeding. Folklore and old wives' tales abound, but factual material is now in abundance, too, thanks to La Leche League,* which has published *The*

* La Leche League International, Inc., 9616 Minneapolis Ave., Franklin Park, Ill. 60131. (*Leche* is the Spanish word for "milk.")

Womanly Art of Breastfeeding and has created an audience for many other good books published on this subject.

We ask our patients to attend La Leche League meetings because they offer (1) a comprehensive course on the various aspects of breastfeeding and (2) companionship with other breastfeeding mothers. What you can learn in a discussion with other mothers is amazing! In fact, that is just how L.L.L. began. The "founding mothers' " discussion of breastfeeding at a picnic turned into group discussion meetings and now has blossomed into a huge international organization. Mothers sharing knowledge is the basis of each meeting. L.L.L. fulfills another fundamental need: you may call your leader (who is an experienced breastfeeding mother with special L.L.L. training) anytime with any problem you are having with your nursing baby. Can you see what a beautiful situation that is? A friend and counselor as close as your telephone.

With L.L.L. set up to handle education for breastfeeding so well, it does make sense that we, who train you for childbirth, wean you to L.L.L. to take over with the second aspect of becoming parents. Duplication of classes is a waste of time and effort, so if there is a local L.L.L., that is where you should be going for information. Frequently childbirth educators are also L.L.L. leaders. Kathy Freese, one of our Denver teachers, leads L.L.L. meetings in her home. If there is no group in your area, you can be instrumental in starting one. At the very least, use *The Womanly Art of Breastfeeding* as a manual. Some of you may reject the "meeting" idea, so it is all in print for you!

Now that I have sold you on the need for L.L.L., let me give you some of the highlights of breastfeeding.

Mother's milk is the natural food for your baby. In these days of dispute over what nutrients are or are not in foods, and what is or is not required, it is very comforting not to have to convert cow's milk into something one hopes is suitable for a human infant. If you eat as well as you know how, your milk will have in it at least everything that your body can supply. Obviously, your good nutrition is important.

When you breastfeed, the baby's milk is always ready. In the middle of the night this is especially pleasant. You need only reach over, take the baby out of the bassinet, and tuck him into your warm bed beside you. Sometimes you both fall asleep and don't wake up until it's time for the next feeding, which is super easy—just turn over and put the baby on the other side! If that idea does not appeal to you, the greatest effort you can put into a night feeding is donning slippers and robe, padding to the nursery, and putting yourself and baby into a rocking chair. In a family that's usually hectic with the activities of small children or busyness of any kind, these moments can be a peaceful communion between the two of you.

I am reminded by Lynn Rimel, another of our Denver teachers of natural childbirth, that there is an added effort at the night feeding—the strong possibility of having a wet (perhaps even smelly) bundle who needs changing before nursing begins. This, of course, is a very usual problem with babies. (Bowel movements of breastfed babies are usually rather loose and much less smelly than if bottle-fed. It could be considered an advantage, I suppose.)

Instant readiness is important at times other than the middle of the night. Feeding is quickly available wherever you are. How easy it is to put baby to breast anytime the slightest bit of fussing begins. Too easy, in fact. You must be wary of using yourself as a pacifier, or you may have your baby snacking all day long and never settling down to his routine. It may discourage you from breastfeeding, too, if you seem to nurse continuously. However, when it is feeding time (established by the baby and not by the clock, usually at approximately three-hour intervals in a very young baby), you have the baby satisfied immediately. If it's "fussy time" for the baby, sometimes only Mommy can make him secure, and that's when your role as pacifier can be used and is permissible.

Breastfeeding can be assisted with one arm, leaving the other free for making peanut butter sandwiches, holding a book as you read to your three-year-old, or just general loving of the other children.

A breastfeeding mother can take her baby with her anywhere very easily. A pediatric psychiatrist in Denver told us at a panel discussion on breastfeeding that she had taken a nursing baby to a formal banquet. One of our graduates, Mrs. Arlene French, was featured in the Denver *Post*, riding her bicycle to Denver University with her baby on her back and taking the baby to classes. No bottles to carry!

The secret of all this "take the baby anywhere" is to have a blouse that easily allows breastfeeding without exposing yourself. No one minds seeing you in a bikini, but try showing any cleavage while breastfeeding your baby and you may face the morality squad. I cannot explain the rationale, but check out Ann Landers' columns and you'll discover frequent entries on the subject. I found it particularly rewarding to nurse a baby in public with no one the wiser (a little game I played). It would occasionally backfire when a stranger came up to admire the baby!

Breastfeeding seems to offer what a baby needs, emotionally as well as nutritionally. Our Rienne is a good example. She likes to hear my stories about how I "wore" her for months. She was either at the breast or on my hip. We moved during that year—no wonder she clung to me. She hated that car ride of half an hour between houses and would scream nonstop unless I nursed her the whole time! I began to worry about the dependent and clinging toddler I would have. She wanted nothing to do with anyone but me. Nursing periods were gradually becoming slightly farther apart—and suddenly, with no other warning, she weaned herself, as though she'd had a plan! As my milk supply did not have an on-off switch, I was in need of her taking just a bit for a day or two following her decision. She was indignant! Not one touch would she give me. Her need had apparently been satisfied and independence is still a dominant factor in her personality. The independence of this child is still a dominant factor in her personality. So what may seem a very dependent nursing baby may end up an independent child. Nursing babies are all different from each other.

Breastfeeding has its physical rewards for the mother, too. It facilitates involution of the uterus, which returns to its normal size more quickly because the baby's sucking causes a simultaneous reflex contraction in the uterus (otherwise known as after-birth pains). Immediate postpartum nursing, while you are still on the delivery table, can help prevent hemorrhage by this very strong contracting.

Our doctors have gained a certain notoriety in Denver medical circles by allowing their patients to nurse the baby on the delivery table. A staff nurse (also our patient) told us this story: One of the obstetricians was having trouble with a mother who had just given birth and was bleeding heavily (it sometimes happens—even in natural childbirth). He told the nurse to get another doctor *fast*. Dr. Bradley happened to be in the hall. He rushed in when called and quickly recognized what was happening. He calmly walked over to where the baby was, forgotten in a corner, picked it up, and put it to the mother's breast. Then he began to help the doctor who was packing the mother's vagina in order to stop the bleeding. The bleeding was soon controlled by the sucking, not the packing. The episode made a believer of one more obstetrician.

According to Karen Pryor in *Nursing Your Baby*,* "This immediate feeding is deeply rewarding to the mother, as well as being physically

---

* Rev. ed. (New York: Harper & Row, 1973), p. 75. Also published by Pocket Books, Inc.

beneficial. The firm contraction of the uterus which results suggests that her intense emotional response to this immediate feeding sets into operation a very strong let-down reflex. The weak and unreliable let-down reflex so typical of many new nursing mothers in the United States may be at least in part a result of delaying the first feeding beyond the critical period."

So the immediate contractions of the uterus are helping the mother both by pulling her uterus back to its normal size and by establishing a good let-down reflex, without which a successful breastfeeding routine cannot easily be established. The let-down reflex allows milk to flow out of the milk glands.

You may frequently hear "But there's no milk at first anyway"; or "The milk comes in on the third day." A fluid called colostrum is present in the breasts even before the baby's birth. It is a highly nutritious, creamy liquid, low in fat and carbohydrate content, easily digested, and it is known to be rich in immunity factors. It has a cleansing effect on the lower digestive tract. Colostrum will be present in the milk for up to ten days.

It has always amazed me how anyone knows when her milk "comes in." The only way to find out is to take a sample in a clear container and look at it—and how does a mother know what human milk looks like? As a matter of fact, it looks very blue and not like "good, rich" milk at all! So appearance is an unreliable yardstick. Sometimes when your milk comes in, your breasts become overfull. Just in case you had triplets, nature is making sure you have enough milk. Or you may become swollen or sore as the milk glands "go into production." They gather all the bodily resources and overdo to the point of discomfort. This lasts only a short time. Having the baby nurse allows the breasts to determine what production is necessary; the milk glands will calm down and produce the right amount of milk for your baby. If the baby is swallowing as he sucks, is having six to eight wet diapers a day—then, whether you have milk or colostrum, does it matter? "When the milk comes in" is a cliché often used but it has little impact on mother or baby as it happens.

Looking back over five breastfeeding experiences, I am amazed to realize what we saved. I saved time by not making formula and sterilizing bottles. We saved money not buying milk for formula. I saved myself for each baby. Instead of "propping" a bottle or letting an older child give the feeding, I sat comfortably rocking my baby with no guilt about things not done, because the baby came first.

The only big disadvantage of breastfeeding is the undeniably self-righteous attitude that we tend to assume. Sometimes it will even tend toward fanaticism. I have always made a supreme effort to hide or cover my feelings, but it is not easy, nor is it always successful. This undoubtedly explains the defensive attitude of some bottle-feeding mothers toward the "Society of Breastfeeders."

I am always impressed by women who know themselves well enough to have a realistic, non-angry reason for not breastfeeding. One woman, whom I admire for her honesty but with whom I can never agree on almost any subject, says, "I could never tolerate such an intimate relationship with anyone." Another very good and loving mother says, "I would feel confined in a breastfeeding situation. I want to know that someone else can care for my baby when I have the need to get away."

I, too, feel the need to get away. Getting away from the children is a legitimate need for mothers. At least once a week my husband treats me to a night out. Often during the day I plan outings with friends. Once breastfeeding is established, it is simple to take the baby with you, but sometimes you need a rest from each other. For an evening out, I would nurse before going and leave a bottle of apple juice or my own expressed milk to be given during my absence. Usually the babies resisted anything so insulting! If they were hungry enough, however, they would take what was offered. It did not seem to hurt them—and I know that I needed that evening out with Richard. The hardest thing to do once you are parents is to have a conversation at home. Too many interruptions!

A trip away from home, if it is only for pleasure, is worth putting off until the baby is no longer nursing. We solved the problem once by taking eight-year-old Joe along with eight-month-old Ritchie and had a wonderful time at Expo '67 in Montreal. It is always a good experience to be able to spend extra time with one or two children. Joe was a big help with the baby, too. We took turns carrying him in a "Snugli"* and considered ourselves one of the exhibits at Expo because of all the attention we drew.

Hard as we breastfeeding mothers try, humility keeps being pushed aside by pride.

It has been proved that allergies can be prevented by breastfeed-

---

* A baby carrier created by the Moores of Evergreen, Colo. For information write: Snugli, Rt. 1, Box 685, Evergreen, Colo. 80439.

ing and a late introduction of other foods (four to six months). There are many studies which show that breastfeeding prolongs babies' natural immunity to infections.

One thing all mothers who have breastfed agree upon is that they become better mothers. It will not turn you into the perfect mother, and maybe you will not even become as good as the lady across the street who prefers the bottle routine, but there is an emotional involvement with your baby that is good. I have many times had to nurse a crying baby when it did not suit me to do so. I had other things planned for that half hour. Once I sat quietly for a few minutes with baby at breast, however, I would forget all those things I thought needed doing.

I remember being furiously, dramatically angry at someone (who and why I can't recall) as I began feeding Allison once when she was tiny. It was therapy for me because my great rage slipped away as I put her to breast. Allison did not seem to have indigestion from it either!

So check your telephone directory for La Leche League meetings, or send for *The Womanly Art of Breastfeeding* and find out all you can about the natural way to feed your baby.

Bust Booster

This exercise will:

1. Strengthen chest muscles that help support the breasts.
2. Help to maintain good shoulder posture.
3. Help when you have heartburn and indigestion.
4. Increase blood flow to the breasts; therefore it may be used later to increase milk supply.

The pectoral muscles help give support to the breasts. Since the breasts become heavier and bigger with pregnancy and breastfeeding, stronger pectorals are indicated.

Breast tissue is mostly fat deposits surrounding the milk-producing glands and covered by skin. There is no muscle in the breast. This means that breast size cannot be increased by exercise. It also means that breast tissue which sags and stretches cannot be rebuilt—since only muscle tissue can be rebuilt. It is necessary, therefore, to prevent sagging and stretching of breast tissue by good support in a bra. If you prefer to go bra-less, I suggest that you develop a good philosophy about sagging breasts!

The extra weight of your breasts, plus the cuddling position which is frequently used for breastfeeding, tend to pull your shoulders down. The breast booster exercise will help strengthen your chest and shoulders to maintain better posture and at the same time relax these overworked muscles.

HOW

1. Sit in a tailor position on the floor. Support each breast with the inside of each bent elbow.

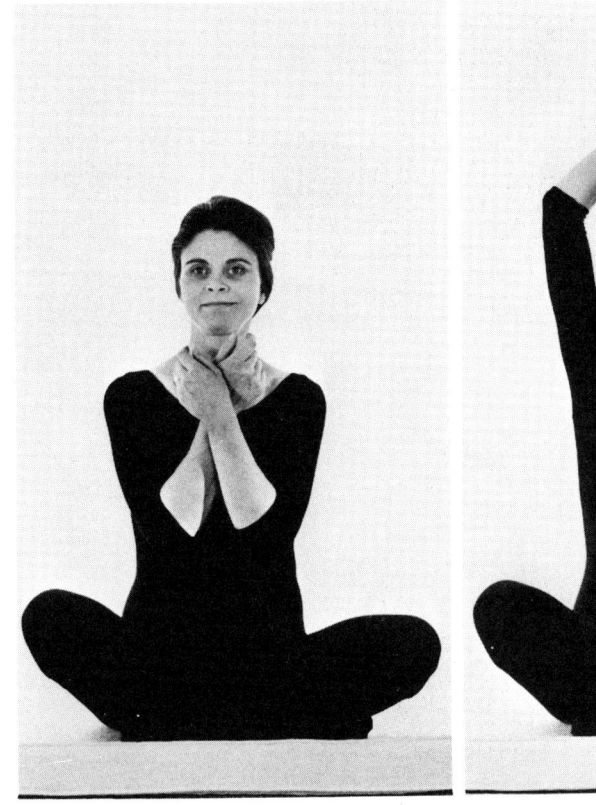

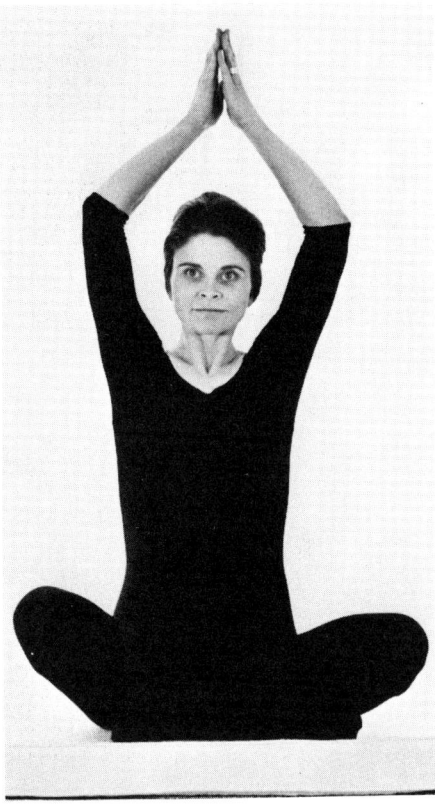

2. Press your arms against your body as you raise your hands above your head. This gently massages your breasts, stimulating circulation.
3. Lower your arms until your hands are below your waist, slightly behind you, with palms up.
4. Now swing the backs of your hands toward each other, behind you, five times (thumbs up).

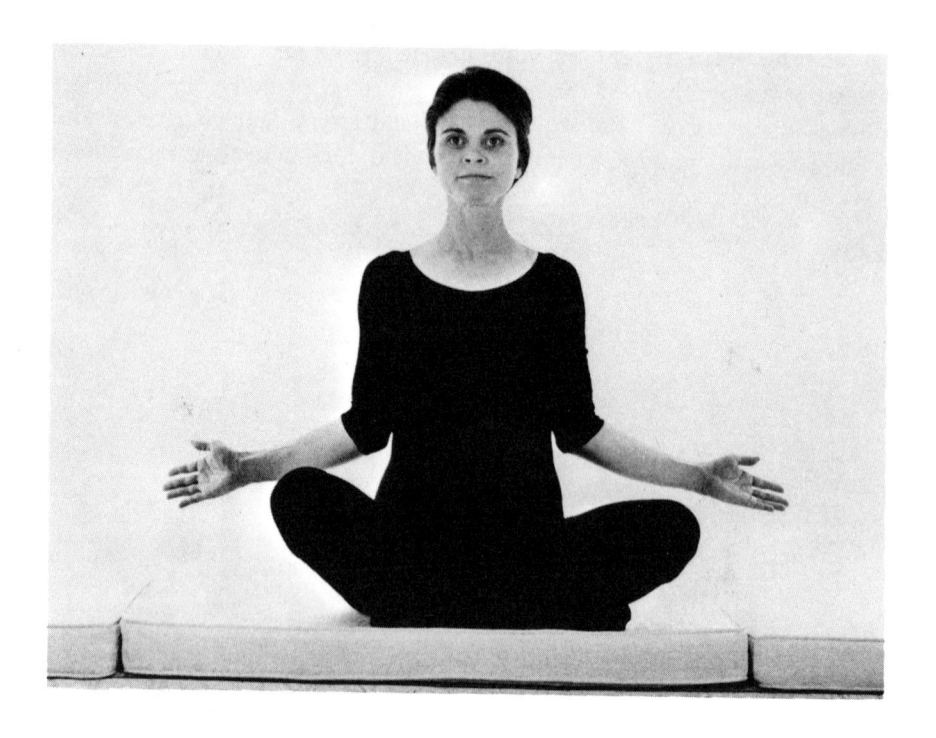

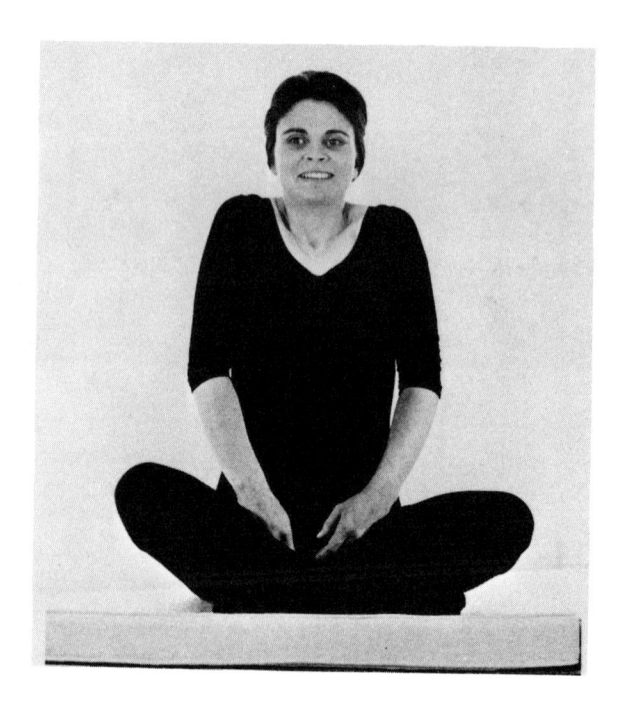

5. Bring your hands to your lap.
6. Take a deep breath while trying to touch your shoulders to your ears.

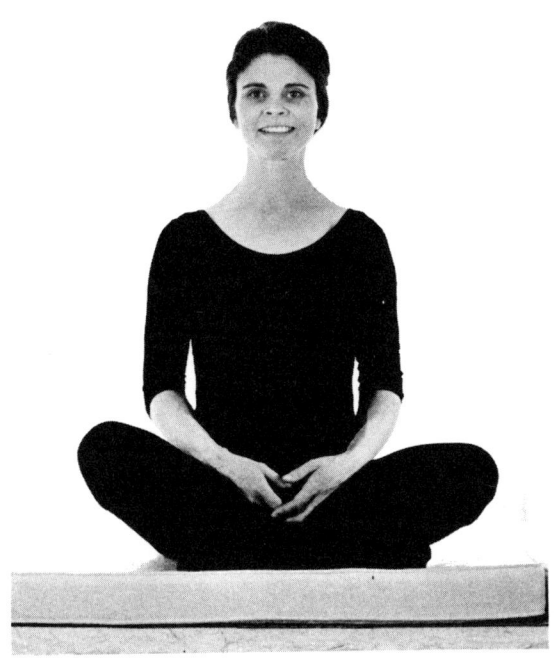

7. Let the breath out and the shoulders drop at the same time, while keeping the breastbone high. It leaves you feeling very good, somewhat invigorated, and with a relaxed upper back.

WHERE Do bust booster in private, on the floor, and always in a tailor sitting position so that your chest muscles do the work instead of your back. There are times when numbers 6 and 7 can be done to relax your shoulders and upper back without going through the whole exercise. You may need a good stretch in church or in the classroom and this can be done rather unobtrusively. Doing the complete exercise in front of others is sure to create a sensation, however.

WHEN *During Pregnancy.* Do bust booster approximately three times a day as a chest muscle exercise and to improve your posture. Do it to relax the upper part of your body. It can also be an effective exercise whenever heartburn distress occurs.

After the Birth. For increasing your supply of breast milk, wait and see if you need to do it. Try to maintain the three times daily to keep muscles in good tone, but if this brings milk rushing out and creates a problem, use a less strenuous chest exercise. If you have a need to create a better milk supply (that is, if the baby seems to demand more milk), then try this to hurry up the process. You will find that it is definitely a help!

Nipple Care

Nothing can be more discouraging to a new mother of a breast-feeding infant than sore nipples. This condition can be prevented by some easy preparation during the last three to four months of pregnancy.

Babies have been categorized according to their sucking, as:

Barracudas—Ouch!
Procrastinators—They sleep for the better part of the first week.
Gourmets—They taste, then smack their lips before beginning.
Resters—Nurse a bit, rest a bit is their way.
Mouthers—These are the babies who do lots of testing without much action.

Any group of nursing mothers could make up its own list of "Games Babies Play." There is the "social nurser," who has to take part in whatever is going on in the room while grasping the nipple in his mouth. This is especially common with older babies. There are the "now I have you to myself" nursers. They fuss and won't eat until Mother is in a quiet room alone with them.

Because of the "barracudas" especially, you should have nipples that can "take it."

We have found from experience that soap and alcohol are unnecessary for cleansing and are very drying to the skin; therefore they should be avoided.

If you live in a dry climate, such as ours in Denver, you need to take extra precautions. We suggest that you use no soap at all and apply lots of oil to your whole body. You may try our method or not, but please use no soap on the nipple area.

You natural-look gals who do not wear a bra will be way ahead on toughening your nipples. From the constant rubbing against clothes, yours will already have lost their tenderness. Topless sunbathing would also be helpful in preparing nipples for breastfeeding. Make sure that you do not have dry and brittle skin. Use a precautionary oil to keep the skin pliable.

I would be concerned, for cosmetic reasons only, about sagging breast tissue if you wear no support during pregnancy and breast-feeding. It is not uncommon to have stretch marks along the sides of the breast, because of the increase in size and weight. I believe that a good support in a brassiere with a comfortable, wide strap over the shoulder is necessary. Make sure the bra is big enough in the cup. You may have to get a series of sizes during your pregnancy. Plenty of care in wearing the proper support and lots of lubrication to the skin during breast-feeding and pregnancy should prevent stretch marks and sagging breasts.

Everyone's skin is different and some of you would have no problem with cracking or bleeding nipples even if you made no preparation. Others will need twice as much preparation as I suggest and still be very tender. How the baby sucks will be another factor. A fairly good indication of skin tenderness is how well you suntan. Girls who tan easily and quickly and never burn will probably have very little trouble toughening their skin for the worst barracuda-type nurser. If, however, you burn easily and tan slowly or poorly, it is an indication that much preparation is needed.

HOW To have soft, rubbery, pliable nipples, use an oily lubricant (anything will do except mineral oil).* You may use vegetable cooking oil, hydrous lanolin, or a cream that you routinely use on your body and know to be good for your skin. Perfumed oils are sometimes irritating to the skin. Lotions containing alcohol are drying. Apply a generous coating all over the breast and on the abdomen, too, to prevent stretch marks. Then grasp the nipple firmly (as in a pinch) and pull. Do ten to twelve times, rotating your hand so that you do not pull in only one spot. Pull out on the whole pigmented area, or areola, and let your fingers slip off the end of the nipple at the completion of each pull. If colostrum is expressed, it can be massaged back into the skin as a lubricant.

While you are doing this ten to twelve times on each breast, run warm water into the bathtub. Climb in for a relaxing soak when you have completed the nipple pulls. The warm water will cleanse you (it's amazing how clean and fresh you can stay with no soap—try it!) and rinse off the excess oil from your body while your warmed skin seems

---

* The American Medical Association urges physicians not to prescribe mineral oil due to its absorption of vitamins and minerals from the body—which are then excreted with the feces. Even with external use there is a risk of absorption.

to absorb more of the oil. Pat yourself dry with a towel—don't rub—and your skin will feel soft but not greasy. You can dress without a sticky feeling, but it is even more comfortable if the whole routine is done just before bedtime.

I found that for the first week or so, this nipple pulling required a diversionary tactic. I was uncomfortable doing it and I felt like an idiot! So: (1) go into the bathroom and bolt the door; (2) don't look in the mirror; (3) have something else to think about. I am a confirmed comics reader. Much of the newspaper I can glance over, but the comics I read carefully. (My father is responsible for teaching me to study each drawing for details.) Obviously, this takes little effort, so I can do it while engaging in nipple pulling. (I do my pelvic rocks while reading the comics, too.) You will be pleasantly surprised to find that after only a few days, the "scrunchy" feeling leaves you and you can do your nipple care without embarrassment or discomfort!

WHERE Probably in private!

WHEN Ten to twelve ouchy pulls each day for the last four months of pregnancy.

CLASS FIVE

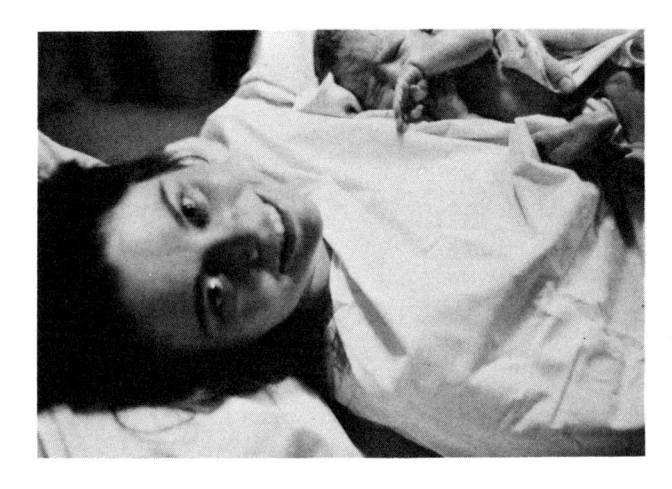

How Labor Feels
Signs of Labor
False Labor
First-Stage Labor
Transition

You are now in your seventh month and your baby is kicking vigorously. He weighs about four pounds and is looking much more like a newborn baby than before. Your baby could very possibly live if born.

Isn't it amazing how quickly the months have gone by? Your baby is becoming more and more a part of you and your husband's lives as a separate personality. He awakens you in the middle of the night because he needs to stretch. You may want to lean into your husband's back and let his baby kick on him for a while. A name for the baby becomes more of a need. I recommend name books for babies as good light middle-of-the-night reading. There are days when every mother is sure she can't wait the many weeks until the baby's arrival. He will surely be easier to handle "out" than "in," you decide. There are other days when you wonder if you can possibly be ready for the baby in time.

Your husband will have settled into his role of prospective father by now. He has usually become aware of his wife's needs better than she knows them herself. It is such a pleasure to be with couples as they anticipate and prepare for this beautiful event in which they will both take part.

Now, too, the realization dawns that it will be up to you, the mother, to allow this increasingly large being to come into the world from the shelter of your body. This acceptance is part of pregnancy and does not seem to occur to you any earlier than necessary. But now you are ready to think about it and we can discuss the actuality of labor.

How Labor Feels

What does labor really feel like? How I wish there were an easy answer to the question. There are as many answers as there are babies. The old smug reply "You'll know when you are in labor" is not at all true. It was harder to know with our fifth baby than with the first, so experience is not always a help either. There are some generalizations and guidelines, however, which will enable you to be pretty sure.

Especially now do we need help from all our class members with experience in childbirth. The hardest part of teaching about labor is that *no two labors are ever the same.*

The most amazing part of early labor for many of you relaxed, prepared, and knowledgeable women is that the contractions are so light and easy and that you are so comfortable. The tales of pain and horror that you have heard make you expect something very difficult. Usually, but not always, labor begins with slow, light contractions, a tensing of the uterus that holds for thirty seconds or less. It may cause you to stop moving because you feel as though you have a heavy weight in your abdomen, but no other sensation. The uterus is very hard and firm and pushed out into the abdomen at this time. When it relaxes, you will go on with what you were doing. Only after several repetitions of this, within a short space of time, will you realize that it could be the beginning of labor. Now you should time the interval from the beginning of one contraction to the beginning of the next to find out how often the contractions are coming. Timing the length of each contraction will be helpful information by the time you get to the hospital, too. (The duration may be thirty to forty-five seconds, maybe even a minute, or more.)

Although it's hard to tell you how labor feels, I must try! You may feel a cramping sensation in the abdomen. Sometimes it begins at the top of the pelvis and moves down. Sometimes it begins in the back and moves around into the abdomen. We've had laboring women who mistook their contractions for a stomachache or called the doctor to ask what to do about flu! Anyone who has experienced menstrual cramps thinks beginning labor is too easy to be the real thing. Some women experience labor in their back only. They get a recurring low backache that lasts a short time, then is gone, then comes again, etc. Sometimes absolutely no sensation is felt until it's time to push. That is more the exception than the rule and could be quite a problem when you think about it—no warning that you are in labor! So you see, there are many variations of how labor contractions *feel!*

Signs of Labor

There are other signs of labor. One is very illusive—the nesting instinct. If you have an urge to do a total spring housecleaning and it is very near your due date—don't! It may be that your body is demonstrating a surge of energy which should be available for labor. Saving energy gets you out of lots of housecleaning, too!

Actual signs of labor are:

- Beginning of contractions
- Breaking of the bag of water
- "Bloody show"

Beginning of contractions. This we've already discussed. Check with your doctor, but a general rule of thumb is to come to the hospital when the contractions are ten minutes apart or less. I once woke up in the night with contractions five minutes apart, so we got ready to go directly to the hospital. I was earlier than I needed to be, but you never know!

How far from the hospital do you live? Should you phone ahead to either the doctor or the hospital? What was your past labor experience, if any, like? What kind of weather is likely? How reliable is your transportation? What will you do with the other children, if any; what could you do as an alternate plan—if Grandma has the flu, who else could take little Dana? If your labor begins during your husband's working hours, will he come home or meet you at the hospital? Who else could drive you to the hospital? (My neighbor offered any help *except* driving me to the hospital if Dick was at work—so better check ahead!)

Find the best route to the hospital and give it a trial run. Consider all these questions now. They are all factors that will seriously affect your peace of mind and therefore your ability to deal with labor. Settle them at once! Plan for all contingencies and arrange suitable alternative plans, then you'll both feel comfortable about your approaching due date.

When your contractions become regular or rhythmical, and about ten minutes apart, wend your way to the hospital—or use your own doctor's criterion if it differs from this. Do what you are told! Even when doctors' orders were followed, babies have been born in the car—not always the most delightful experience and rather hard on the upholstery.

If you live in an out-of-the-way region and are concerned about not making it to the hospital in time, I suggest two things: First, have a serious, frank discussion with your doctor and let him help you solve your problem. Secondly, Dr. Gregory White has written a small, easily understood book called *Emergency Childbirth*.* Read it and acquaint yourself with the procedure. If you've done neither of these things, here's an easy rule to remember: Do not cut anything. Put the baby to breast with skin-to-skin contact between mother and baby. Bundle them up warmly and then contact your doctor! Do not do anything about the placenta and the cord. Nature has a way of dealing with these which in most cases is perfect. As long as the baby is at breast, nature's method is at work. But you will be very relieved to have your doctor walk in and take over, I can assure you!

Better to get to the hospital on time and enjoy the security that it affords. You can concentrate on what you are doing there.

Breaking of the bag of water. As you know, the baby is floating in salt water enclosed in a membranous balloon called the amniotic sac. The amount of this colorless liquid varies, as does the toughness of the membrane. This accounts for the spontaneous rupture of membranes sometimes prematurely, sometimes during labor, and sometimes, rarely, not breaking at all. Some babies are born with sac fluid and all intact. In the latter case, the sac must be broken quickly so that the baby can breathe. Superstition claims that a baby born in a caul, as it is called, is truly gifted and will live an outstanding life. Abraham Lincoln, for one, is supposed to have been born in a caul.

So the membrane has to break sometime. It may break early in labor—even before the onset of contractions. It may break during labor. Or the doctor may break it as your labor progresses to speed up

---

* Franklin Park, Ill.: Police Training Foundations, 1958.

contractions.* Sometimes the membrane breaks several weeks early, in which case the doctor will have to induce labor—that is, use medical means to bring it on. Generally, a baby should be born within forty-eight hours after the bag of water breaks, as any longer time makes possible an infection, which endangers the lives of both mother and infant.

How does it feel when the bag of water breaks? There is no sensation other than warm fluid between your legs. Tightening hard on your Kegel muscle helps control it somewhat but not completely. The liquid is colorless and varies in amount. It did not stain my blue armchair! You may spill only a cup or so—or you could have gallons (well, it seems that much!). Ordinarily, as long as you are standing or walking, the baby's head will act as a cork pushed into a bottle, and only little dribbles will escape. If you are lying in bed as your bag of water breaks, you have a much better likelihood of a flood.

We all worry about inundating the supermarket or filling a church pew with amniotic fluid! Usually, the amount is too small to affect others. If anyone around you does realize what has happened, the reaction is always one of wanting to help. You will probably have fifteen offers to drive you to the hospital, take your groceries home, and keep your children. Childbirth is exciting to us all.

Once the membrane breaks, you'll probably have to use a towel between your legs to absorb the fluid when you move about.

Our rule is to go directly to the hospital when your bag of water breaks. The doctor must check you immediately to assure the safety of the baby. Ask your doctor what he wants you to do if this happens. Generally, labor will begin within a few hours, if it has not already begun. When the membrane ruptures, the baby will be born within forty-eight hours in most cases, by medical induction if necessary.

"Bloody show." This is always present in hard labor and all medically trained persons are familiar with it. Sometimes you will see bloody show early in labor, or even before you know that labor is beginning. In this case, it is an indication that you are dilating and the mucus that has plugged the cervix—the lower end of the uterus—forming a seal, is beginning to come away as the cervix starts to open. Some-

* There are studies done by Dr. Roberto Caldeyro-Barcia of Montevideo, Uruguay, which show that the amniotic sac filled with fluid equalizes the tremendous pressure of the uterine contraction so that the baby's head does not receive the full stress. It proves that intact membranes have a definite value.

times it is just a heavy, egg-whitelike vaginal discharge, but it may become streaked or tinged with blood and may, indeed, even look very bloody to you. This, then, is "bloody show." Here again, check with your own doctor for his rules. Our rule of thumb is that if there is more blood than a normal menstrual flow, then hurry to the hospital. Bleeding is *not* normal in labor and indicates a serious problem which must be dealt with immediately. Show is perfectly normal and can be taken casually. Your problem is to know the difference. I suggest that if you are at all unsure, get to the hospital, where help is available. Take no chances!

If bloody mucus, or "bloody show," precedes labor, sit at home and wait for labor to begin before rushing to the hospital.

False Labor

"False labor," rare though possible with first babies, and rather common for all subsequent labors, is a series of uterine contractions which do not continue on to the birth of the baby. You may consider that the uterine muscle is having a practice session. There are contractions all through your pregnancy, though you may not be aware of them. They become noticeable as you get closer to your due date. Usually they are spasmodic and come one at a time. You may be able to cause a contraction by reaching to your top cupboard shelf or by lifting your two-year-old. They are usually referred to as Braxton Hicks contractions. In false labor, on the other hand, the contractions continue for an extended period at a regular rate. You may cause it by overexertion, or by a particularly strenuous day. I would guess that the Christmas season gives rise to an increase in false labor.

True labor does not respond or change with your activity. It almost always continues at a regular rate no matter what you do. False labor, on the other hand, will change as your activities change, then will become very irregular, and eventually will stop.

What can you do to tell the difference between false and true labor? You do something quite opposite to what you were doing when contractions began. If you wake at night with contractions and you have reason to doubt that it's the real thing (for instance, it is several weeks before your expected date, or you may have been having lots of activity of the uterus which has not amounted to labor), then get up and move around the house a bit. Time your contractions. A ten-minute shower or warm bath is another good way to test. If the contractions continue at a fairly even rate, you are *not* in false labor! If it is false labor the contractions will slow down and stop and you can go back to bed.

If you are very busy getting dinner ready for ten guests, feeding the children, and trying to bed them down before the guests arrive, were up late the night before making beef Burgundy and sewing a new party dress because you had nothing to wear, and have spent all this day cleaning the house—this is a perfect time for contractions to begin! You must relax and give your uterus a chance to stop being irritated by all your activity. A warm bath or shower would be a good test now. Then lie down for a few minutes. Chances are it's false labor and the contractions will gradually fade out. If they don't, I hope those ten dinner guests are good friends and can have the party by themselves. At least there will be someone to stay with the children!

It can be embarrassing to go to the hospital and have everything stop and have to go home again, but it's a common error. Doctors generally admit laughingly that most of them have taken their wives to the hospital in labor, only to be told that it was false. I've yet to hear any female M.D.'s statistics on their own labors, but they undoubtedly are not always right either. The point is—don't be embarrassed. It's hard to know if you are in false labor or true. You might just as well be safe and get to the hospital.

First-Stage Labor

A visit to the obstetrics ward of the hospital is an important prerequisite of Class Five. In our case, the hospital sets up tours and schedules for our patients. If your teacher gives you the tour, then it may be the same evening as Class Five is held. You should be shown the admitting procedure, the labor room, and the necessary routine that is followed—a discussion of shave and enema, if required, where your clothes will be stored, what forms are to be filled out and signed, where you are allowed to walk and where not (there may be hours of walking time ahead!).

Ask questions and find out about details that bother you. That's what the tour is for. You will be shown the delivery room, how the table adjusts, where the baby is placed after birth, the mirror, where your husband is to sit. Then you will be shown the recovery room, and finally a room typical of one where you'll be until discharge from the hospital.

The tour is to dispel any questions or fears you have, so feel free to ask questions.

In our hospital we have a piece of plywood with ten holes of progressive sizes drilled into it. The smallest is one centimeter and the largest is ten centimeters. Each time you are checked by a nurse or doctor for cervical dilation, you can be shown your size on the chart. When you are 5 cm, you see that you're about midway in the progression. You should realize that usually the first half of the first stage takes longer than the second half of the first stage. In other words, it takes the uterus longer to open the cervix to 5 cm than it does to open it from 5 cm to 10 cm—considered complete dilation.

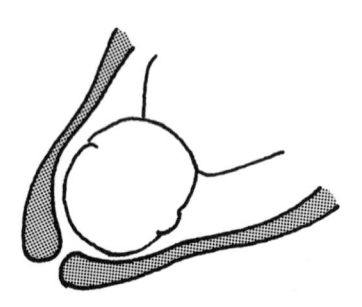

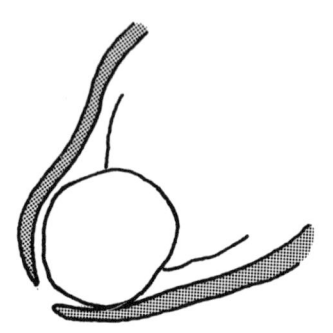

Effacement or thinning

The other measurement that is needed to check your progress in labor is effacement or thinning. The cervix does not open like the neck of a bottle, but rather like a turtleneck sweater. As the walls of the cervix thin out to become stretched tight over the baby's head, then dilation of the opening of the cervix will be much faster.

Let's consider that you have been admitted to the hospital and have gone through all the necessary procedures. You and your husband may now walk the corridors of the obstetrics ward while you go through the early stages of dilating. (Be sure to find out on the hospital tour where you may walk. If you are lucky, you'll be allowed to walk by the nursery window.) As the dilations and thinning progress, however, and it becomes uncomfortable walking, it is time to return to your room.

When a contraction begins, you will bend slightly forward and rest your arms against your husband. Your uterus can fall forward and will be more comfortable. You are the one who will decide when it's time to get into bed so that you can relax completely and breathe abdominally with each contraction. Be sure to be in the side-lying relaxation position that we practiced in classes. There is often a clock on the wall so you can time your contractions. Your husband may even be writing them down. It is helpful to get relaxed and loose and begin abdominal breathing fifteen to twenty seconds before you expect a contraction. You get a head start! When the contraction is over you can wiggle and move about or sit up and continue your card game or your conversation with your husband. Your activities between contractions will change as your labor progresses. The harder and closer together the contractions are, the less likely you are to need anything to do. Remember to move your arms and legs, though, so you won't have them "falling asleep."

Your husband will have his real test of love at this time. The more work relaxing is, the more you need him. If he can be very vocal, it is a help. He can whisper relaxing and encouraging things in your ear. If that is hard for him, have him read my quieting poem, or some other written piece that helps you stay relaxed. One couple had a super system: to relax his wife he sang ballads to his own guitar accompaniment. Not all of us have husbands with that particular talent, but they are all talented in knowing how they can help the woman they love.

Back rubbing is another act of love. Many husbands perform heroic feats of arm strength in this way. One easy and comfortable way to apply pressure is to press the palm of his hand against the tailbone area (lower back) where it feels best to you. It's easier on your skin and may even feel better than rubbing.

Each night, as you prepare for bed, you should rehearse together. Pretend that you are having a contraction and let your husband practice his skills at relaxing you and seeing that your abdominal breathing is very slow and deep. You will have lots of clowning and laughing, but what a difference when you are really in labor! You've found out what works and do not have to waste time and effort figuring it out. You can give helpful suggestions when you practice. Your husband can learn to avoid the ticklish spots and can leave out irritating words. You may like his hand on your abdomen as a reminder with your breathing. You may like a soft touch here and there to help you loosen parts of your body. You may like an idea of how long the contraction has been going —"It's thirty seconds now, halfway through," or whatever. Practice together. If he is really a coach, he won't wait until final game time to begin working with the star player. No athlete wins laurels without a coach, working very hard.

Another aspect of your husband's being a strong coach in labor is that it shows immediately to the hospital staff. They realize that this is a couple who know what they are doing. You'll probably get lots of cooperation. If you are trying to prove a point at your hospital, this is the way to do it.

Transition

Now we have come to the end of the first stage of labor and we call it transition. You are dilated between seven and ten centimeters. Transition (and first stage) will be over when you begin to push—and that means you will be in second-stage labor.

Remember, we relax completely and breathe abdominally with each contraction in first stage. You've been doing just that until now. You are becoming better at it all the time and it is what will keep you comfortable through transition. Transition is the hardest part of labor, but it is also the shortest part.

We can divide you into three groups according to the way you will experience transition:

1. Some of you will never know you went through it. You were 7 cm dilated one minute and your cervix dilated completely with the very next contraction. Your uterus did the work too quickly for you to be aware of it. Suddenly you are ready to push.

2. Some of you will be working so hard at relaxing that you will not be aware of anything but a gradual increase in intensity of your labor. After the baby is born, and you and your husband are reminiscing, you'll be able to recognize where it was that your transition took place.

3. Then there is the third group. Everything gets messed up! You need a good understanding of transition so that you don't become discouraged and "give up" and you need strong support to maintain your relaxation. Your husband will earn a trophy for coaching you through. For you in the third group, here's an explanation of transition:

During transition, the uterus does its most difficult, most violent work. It is contracting very hard and rather quickly. Sometimes contractions will come as close together as one minute and last almost as long. Sometimes the intervals will increase in length during this time, however.

The uterus, as it squeezes into a hard contraction, forces most of the blood out of itself (not the baby) and into your body. This means you have nearly half again as much blood pushed into your circulatory system as your body normally carries. (The increase was to care for the pregnant uterus.) So while you are relaxing with a contraction, you are also feeling very hot and flushed. Your husband may notice that you appear to be blushing. You become uncomfortably warm and wish that you could have the blanket off your bed. Every capillary in your body has extra blood in it and this makes your nerve endings very irritable indeed—so as your husband rubs your back and puts his hand on your tummy to coach your breathing, you feel a distinct desire to hit him in the teeth. Even the nightgown and bed covers are irritating. All these unpleasant sensations—while you are working so hard at relaxing and breathing abdominally with a very hard contraction!

Ah! Now the contraction is ending and you can take care of these unpleasant circumstances. But wait—things are changing. All that blood racing around in you is needed by the uterus again to get ready for its next contraction. Blood rushes back to fill those large veins and arteries in a momentarily loose uterus. Suddenly you feel rather light-headed and dizzy. Not a bad sensation, but it makes you forget to get ready for the next contraction. Oh, dear, that pizza you ate before you knew you were in labor is getting very restless. Perhaps you'll have to give it up, as your body can't have a baby and digest a meal all at the same time. If you do throw up, it's inconsequential compared to the other things you are doing just now! Now what? You are trembling. You're not cold but your body is acting as though you are shivering. The obvious solution is to add an extra blanket. Poor labor coach. If you've been able to give verbal commands as fast as things are happening in your body, he'll think you've lost your mind!

Now you begin another contraction and the whole cycle repeats itself. Well, not quite—you will not vomit more than once, if that.

Fortunately, you've practiced very hard at relaxing and your husband is offering encouragement and lots of verbal energy. Before you know it, you may feel as though you need to have a bowel movement. That is an indication that the baby is low enough to be pressing against the rectum and that second stage has begun. Or you may take a nice, big abdominal breath and then not want to let it out. You may even begin grunting. These are all signs of second stage labor.

Looking back over five labors, I have developed a composite picture of transition, by far the most unique stage of labor. It was the hardest part, requiring every ounce of energy and control I had. I have tried every gimmick I ever read of in a book or heard from any teacher I've met. I always come back to abdominal breathing and total relaxation as the best relief in transition.

In transition I would get very restless and run to the bathroom between contractions. Of course, I got caught there with a contraction more than once! What you find out as you are on your hands and knees on the bathroom floor with a hard-as-a-rock uterus is that it hurts a lot, but it only lasts about one and one-half minutes. Then you can get back to bed and really be ready for the next contraction. We all have to learn to appreciate the effectiveness of what we are doing.

Transition brings on a psychological change, too. I was, all at once, this angelic creature giving birth—a madonna in touch with Creation. I lay in shining light and was above all others—and why in the blankety-blank was my husband not coaching me properly? Who does he think he is to put his head down on his arms to rest at a time like this? Ring for the nurse—get me the doctor—I do not want to be ignored!

I can laugh now, but nothing's funny then. I hope I'm giving you enough warning so that you'll be able to deal with this very short time in your labor. Don't let a few minutes ruin the next wonderful stage. If you give up and need anesthesia now, you'll not be in control and will be unable to enjoy pushing. Pushing is a joy!

Think of your labor as a freight train. Each boxcar is a separate entity. It is joined securely to the cars on either side and all are needed to make a train—but some might be empty or even need to be put off on a siding and left behind. It changes the train very little. All your contractions are linked together to form labor, but if you mess up one or two, it's not the ruin of your whole labor. You've a time between contractions to get yourself together again and be ready. Give yourself a pat on the back for the contractions you handle well and forget the ones you flubbed. No woman alive is going to be perfect with every single contraction in labor. I know from experience that we berate ourselves for the bad, but please praise yourself for the good instead!

You have a month now to work hard at developing a good technique for perfect teamwork with your coach. Do your homework!

CLASS SIX

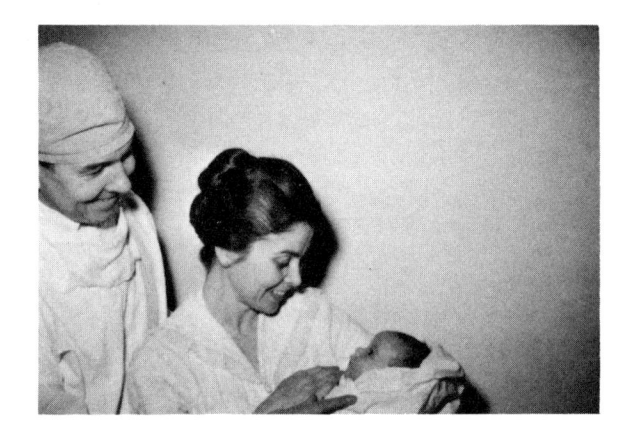

Second-Stage Labor
Birth
First Breastfeeding
Recovery Room
Hospital Stay
Going Home
Review

You have six weeks or less till your due date. Your baby is a real live being now with every part intact and would live if born, though it would be very scrawny and thin, five to five and one-half pounds and 18 inches long. The last two months are important to the growth and development of the baby. At full term the baby weighs six to nine pounds, is about 20 inches long and very active.

Your lives are geared to the birth of the baby. All projects are either cleared up before or put off until after the due date. It's actually a super time for getting things done. Being a deadline, it requires organization.

These last few weeks can seem interminable if you just stop everything and wait. Keep your lives moderately busy and exciting so that the time moves along easily. Do not overcrowd your time and make a haggard, tired mother for labor! Be sure you lie down for a rest at least once a day. Use the elevated position from Class Three more often now. Varicose veins could be a problem, so get your legs up as much as ten minutes every hour for painful, aching legs. It's O.K. to feel very pregnant and to act it! You may be uncomfortable squatting, so do it only when you have to reach to the floor for some reason. That's why you worked so hard to do it well and often earlier in your pregnancy. Now you can do it less often. Lifting and bending may cause a contraction of the uterus—so don't feel guilty about asking someone to help you with things. Your husband won't mind lifting your toddler and your toddler can bend over to "pick things up for Mommy." Just remember you are already carrying at least twenty extra pounds around with you constantly and you won't be ashamed if you are not anxious to do much extra! Your pelvic rock and tailor sit will make life far more comfortable. Do your abdominal breathing and relaxing extra times during the day—it's a good rest as well as practice.

Your sex life in these last weeks deserves a word or two. Most doctors now agree that there is no great risk of infection from so normal a part of your life. You may find that your lovemaking creates contractions of the uterus. This is perfectly normal and only indicates the irritability of muscles getting ready for labor. Pelvic rocking both before and after lovemaking will aid your comfort. Sometimes the pregnant woman is just too big, has too much pressure, and the baby is too low for her to be interested in intercourse. Husbands, be understanding, and realize that she still needs to feel loved, cuddled, and told how wonderful she is. Boy, oh, boy, does she need it! It's not easy to feel confident when you feel awkward.

Remember, every pregnancy is different! Some of you will feel beautiful, graceful, sexy, and your love life will be fantastic. Perhaps the next pregnancy—same couple—will be the opposite. It can be a warm, fulfilling, happy, loving time in your lives, in spite of any limitations in your sex life, if you'll be understanding of each other's needs. You'll have a stronger, better marriage from this shared experience. You'll learn a lot more about each other and yourselves. Be loving. Be kind.

Second-Stage Labor

Now let's begin our last class and discuss second-stage labor.
Once your labor reaches the end of transition, which is the end

of first stage, a major change takes place. It feels very different and *you* act differently.

Second stage means the cervix is fully dilated to allow the presenting part of the baby, usually the head, to come into the vagina or birth canal. Now the passive first stage is over for you. The second stage is usually shorter than the first stage (note—I did not say *always* shorter). Second stage is a time for strenuous activity and total involvement with the work going on inside you. Rather than trying to keep out of the way of the working uterus, as in first stage, now you will make your strong pushes coincide with the effort of the uterus, so second stage will be as efficient as possible.

How do you know when it's time to push? Again, an uncertain answer is what I must give you. There is a variety of reactions that you could experience. Some of you will be absolutely sure that you are in second stage and will begin pushing despite your husband's great efforts to calm you down. *He* doesn't know that you are ready to push, and has become so very good at relaxing you by this time that he may be upset when you refuse to do what he says. He reminds you to relax but you begin holding your breath and bearing down. If you have no doubt that it's pushing time, go ahead and push, but for heaven's sake tell the nurse and/or doctor what you are doing. As Dr. Bradley says, "Push the bell first and your bottom second."

Some of you may be much less certain that it's time to push, but you think it is. Try to relax while you get the doctor or nurse to make sure that you are fully dilated. Pushing too early will slow down the process some, as it causes an edema of the tissue and hardens that lovely soft cervix. So if in doubt, get a professional opinion. Or wait until you really can't avoid pushing.

Some of you may never have a subjective urge to push and will need coaching (remember, there are no "normals" in labor). You may valiantly carry on with your relaxing even though it is not very effective any longer.

You may be aware of a change but not an urge to push. This is where the nurses or doctor will be of great help. They can usually sense the change in your breathing or your attitude and can check your dilation to verify their feelings. Your labor coach undoubtedly sensed the change, too, but without experience may not have known what it meant. Our friends Hesham and Anna Baghdady had this experience. Anna mistook the beginning of labor for "gas pains." Hesham was wise enough to bring her to the hospital—just in case, as quite a few hours had gone by. As they were being admitted to the hospital, Anna was sure that she was a "failure" because she was so lousy at relaxing. A few minutes later, the doctor discovered that she was well into second-stage labor—and she thought she was doing badly! Once told to push, she did magnificently and soon gave birth to a baby boy. As the three of them walked out of the delivery room, she looked up at her husband and said, "Well, honey, what else shall we do today?"

At this point I must talk to the primipara (first-time mother, often abbreviated "primip") separately from the multipara (who has already given birth to one or more). The reason for this is that the first birth will take longer in second stage than subsequent births. The birth canal is a much less muscular area than the uterus. Therefore, once the birth canal has been pushed open and stretched by a normal-size baby, it will allow a baby through more easily the next time. Since the uterus is all muscle, it can tighten up to complete strength so your second labor *could* have a longer first stage than the first labor—though it's usually slightly shorter. Second or third babies may have longer or shorter first-stage labors, but the second stage of labor will usually be shorter than with the first baby. How well you push will make a difference, of course. Other variants could be a tired mother, a large head, the baby's position, and a premature birth, to mention a few. We have more exceptions than rules!

Generalizing, then, if this is your first baby, you'll be left in your labor room bed to push until the baby is closer to the opening of the vagina (or farther down the birth canal). You will be more comfortable on the bed than on the hard, narrow delivery table. You can roll the head of the bed up nearly to a sitting position so that you are in an "almost squat" position for pushing. Between contractions you will lean back into the contour shape of the bed and rest. As a contraction begins, you will take two preparatory breaths and let them out fully. With the third full breath, pull your knees apart and toward your shoulders, hold your breath, and with chin to your chest, bear down with all your strength. If it hurts, you aren't working hard enough. The hard, steady pushing obliterates all other sensations in your perineum and abdomen. Think strong! Push as hard and as long as you are able until you can no longer hold your breath. Release your chin from your chest (raise your head, in other words), let your breath out completely, and if you still feel some contraction in the uterus, take another huge breath, chin to chest, pull legs out and back, and keep pushing. You'll *know* if you try to stop pushing too early. That contraction will be very apparent without your pushing pressure. It's almost too amazing to believe until you try it, but it works!

You will be pushing in bed while your husband changes to his "bunny suit" or "coaching uniform"—whatever your hospital requires him to wear in the delivery room. The doctor will be here by now, we hope, and he will change to his required garb, too. About the time your baby's head begins to be visible as you push—"Caput is showing"—the nurses will move you (sometimes bed and all, sometimes by a cart) to the delivery room.

Back to the "multip" who is ready to push. As soon as you said you had to push, everybody went wild. Your baby could arrive with only two pushes and it's considered a "failure" of the staff if you should have your baby in bed! More comfortable for you, and the baby can fall only two inches to a soft mattress, but most hospitals are extremely conscientious about having the baby arrive into a sterile world. The doctors have been trained to deliver babies while sitting on a stool at the foot of a delivery table and they seem to lack grace and dexterity when reaching over the foot of a bed. I've never heard of a baby suffering from a birth in bed, but most hospitals are determined you shall be on that hard, narrow table. I'm sure the doctor can explain the necessity, whereas I can only think of the difference in comfort. Be that as it may, the nurses will rush you to the delivery room. You may have a contraction as you are moved along the hall—push with it. You will be extremely uncomfortable when you do not push with a contraction. It will make you sympathetic to all those friends who were not taught to push.

Now you are all, multips and primips alike, in the delivery room. I should remind you here that primips *can* have as fast a pushing stage as multips and will be taken immediately to the delivery room. You have become acquainted with it on your hospital tour, so the gleaming walls, huge light, resuscitator, and table of sterile instruments are all old stuff to you. When you get on the delivery table, the leg holders will be put in position and then you can rest your legs in them between pushes. During a push, always get into the squat posture, with legs pulled out and back, chin on chest. As soon as the doctor is in his place with you, the end of the table is lowered so that your bottom is at the edge of it (the same idea as the examining tables in the doctor's office). The doctor will put sterile sheets around you so that he has a sterile (as clean as possible) area for the birth of the baby. Your doctor will explain to you where you mustn't put your hands. Some hospitals are relaxing these rules, realizing that the mother and baby cannot be all that harmful to each other! It is a relatively small matter to you as long as you are allowed to push properly to give birth to your baby.

As the doctor is organizing his end, your husband-coach is on his little stool (the anesthetist's) at your head.

One thing more and you are in complete readiness for pushing. Get the table tilted so that your head is up. Every delivery-room table is made to tilt, and with the doctor's permission, your husband could do it. (The control is at the head of the table.) If you are all agreed, a forty-five-degree angle is optimum for pushing. This affords a downhill slide for the baby, allowing gravity to help you with your pushing. You open the birth canal most effectively in this position. It is also easier to push.

With each push, begin by taking two breaths and letting each one out. As you take your third breath, which you will hold, pull your knees apart and toward your shoulders, holding firmly with your wrists under your knees so you can't slip out of position. Bear down firmly and steadily, with your chin to your chest. Your husband has his arm around your shoulders, helping you keep your back bowed, and is verbally coaching and encouraging you all the time.

Gary and Sue McCutcheon, who teach as a team, have a wonderful training for parents. Gary puts Sue in this position and demonstrates his verbal coaching for the class to hear. "Put your chin down, hold your breath, push hard, relax the Kegel muscle, push hard, that's a girl, you're doing good, keep it up, push hard, keep pushing, make sure you're relaxing that baby door, the baby is coming, we'll soon have a baby, good girl, you're doing well, keep pushing," etc. He keeps this up at a fast, enthusiastic pace as though he were actually a coach of a foot race, spurring on the contestant. As Sue says, who could help but do a good job with that kind of encouragement! In their classes they have each couple practice this out loud and insist on lots of repetition at home. It's the best idea I've heard, and I urge you to do it, too. The coach can be the most important member of the team. His good coaching can make all the difference. How proud you'll be of your teamwork *and* your baby!

As you are doing this hard, efficient pushing, the doctor is watching your perineum to see how well the skin is stretching. When the skin becomes very shiny, tight, and white, it will tear if nothing is done. Since a cut heals better than a rip, his judgment will usually be to do an episiotomy. We do a "midline" episiotomy almost routinely when one is needed at all. That is, the cut is made straight back from your vaginal opening. This is much more comfortable in healing, does less damage to the perineum, and especially to the Kegel muscle, since this is where the sides of muscle are joined together. The baby's head is now "crowning" —pushing hard against the skin of your perineum and even causing it to bulge. The outer tissues, including the skin, are tough and hard to stretch. This is partly the nature of the skin and partly due to our maintaining a constant covering here. During pregnancy, you can prepare this area by using lots of oil, very little soap, no panties, and constant tailor sitting, "Kegeling," and squatting. You will increase the elasticity of the perineum. The cut is always done without even a local anesthetic. There is a natural numbness with the baby's head crowning and with your very hard pushing. The doctor will cut during a contraction and while you are pushing. With that same contraction, the baby's head will be born.

There are two reasons for not giving any kind of anesthetic now. First, you do not feel any pain, so why administer a "painkiller"? To give an anesthetic (even a local), the doctor must slow down the labor by having the mother stop pushing, which is impossible and painful. He would create the pain by giving the remedy. Also, any anesthetic, even a local, may be absorbed by the baby. In a few seconds that very powerful adult dose of relaxant would be in your baby when he needs all his energies for beginning life!*

A local anesthetic will be needed for episiotomy repair. The natural numbness created by your pushing and the head's crowning will be gone by then. When the baby is born and the cord is clamped, the anesthetic will be no threat.

Sometimes an episiotomy is not needed. The doctor will not automatically cut you; he will make a medical decision in each case. Occasionally you may be asked to pant like a puppy for a short time, to allow the skin a chance to stretch slowly over that last fullness of the baby's head.

Birth

As the doctor is making his decision on whether or not to give you an episiotomy, you may be conscious of a very tight stretched feeling in the perineum or specifically at the rectum. You may become aware of the incision the doctor makes only by a release of this pressure, but

---

* Bowes, Brackbill, Conway, and Steinschneider, *The Effects of Obstetric Medication on Fetus and Infant.*

that is a pleasant awareness. Now your baby's head will be born. This is the moment of birth for the mother. Your work is done, and a flood of joy, accomplishment, and love overwhelms you.

Sometimes the contraction is over as the head is born so the baby's body is still in the birth canal. This is a strange feeling for the mother and a rather anxious moment for the father, as he doesn't feel he has a baby until he knows if it is a boy or a girl. Now you must wait patiently for two to three minutes until the next contraction allows you to push the body of your child into the world. (Obviously, a breech baby will not happen this way, and *would* be born in one push.) The doctor has suctioned the mouth and nose and sometimes the baby cries before being completely born. Some doctors will help you to reach down and lift the baby out of the birth canal yourself as soon as the shoulders have been delivered. The closer you can get to your baby, the better!*

With the last push, the father-coach will be standing on tiptoes to determine the sex of his baby. Then the rafters ring with his announcement. Very often your big, strong he-man coach will have tears streaming down his face while he laughs with joy and accomplishment and pride! He's proud of his child, himself, the doctor, and especially his wife. You, the mother, on the other hand, have become maternal in an instant. You beam at your husband, smile tenderly at his masculine tears, kiss any part of him you can reach, his hand, his sleeve, his lips when offered! And you reach for your baby and coo and talk baby talk to this funny little bundle.

Meanwhile, the doctor has been enjoying your reactions in his paternal manner as he has wiped the baby off—prettying it up a bit—suctioned nose and mouth, held it down lower than your body until the cord stopped pulsing (indicating that all the blood belonging to the baby has gone into its little body), clamped and cut the cord, and at last put the baby to your breast.

First Breastfeeding

It is truly amazing that some babies will suck as though really hungry. Only a few minutes old and acting like a pro! Other babies are less interested, but all will nuzzle and search for the nipple. Touch your

* Doris Haire, "The Cultural Warping of Childbirth," in *International Childbirth Education Association News*, vol. II, no. 1, 1972.

baby's cheek and watch the reaction. He immediately turns to that side with mouth open. They are born with that automatic reflex to find food. As your nipple becomes erect from the baby's touch, your uterus will contract and help the placenta to be expelled and the lining of the uterus to remain tight. A tight, hard, contracted uterus will prevent excessive bleeding.

It is about this time that the doctor will inject a local anesthetic into the edges of your episiotomy, if you had one, or your tear if that happened. When the local has made you numb, he'll begin to embroider you together. During this time, the placenta may be expelled. This is called the third stage of labor and may require a push from you. A wait of up to thirty minutes is perfectly normal for the placenta to be delivered. Having the baby at breast usually facilitates the third stage.

When all these details have been completed, you'll be padded (there will be considerable bloody vaginal discharge) and allowed to sit up. Iced orange juice is the reward we give at this time. The parents and the doctor, too, need something to increase their blood sugar after all the energy that has been used in the past few hours. Sometimes it's been a long time since a meal! You can call it a toast to the new baby.

Recovery Room

If the labor was a normal one, and the mother and doctor agree, you may now walk out of the delivery room to your bed. Many hospitals have a recovery room where you'll be put to bed for one or two hours. You will be watched very carefully for blood pressure, pulse, and bleeding. The nurse will check the tightness of your uterus and if it loosens, she'll "knead" it into a tight contraction again (not comfortable but necessary). Sometimes you will be given an ice bag to put on your tummy to help the process. It is important that your uterus remain firm, so you can help by massaging it.

Hopefully, the baby will be left with you throughout as much of this period as possible. There is increasing evidence that these immediate moments after birth are important to the baby. The stimulus of your touch is important to even his breathing and heartbeat. Much is happening in that tiny being, and the closeness to you, the mother, can help it to be smooth and easy. During the first two hours try to cuddle, stroke, and love your baby all you can.

For these two hours, you will be very excited. You want to shout to the world about your new baby. Your husband will brag about you, how well you did, how beautiful you are, how sweet the baby is.

It's especially fun to phone the grandparents to announce the new arrival. No one will believe that you could have just had a baby and sound so well and happy. Our society has warped this whole business of childbirth. It's our privilege to change society!

After two hours of excitement, hyperactive laughing and talking, holding and admiring the baby, trying to breastfeed, phoning friends and relatives to share your news, being moved from one hospital room to another, being terrifically hungry and finally getting some food to eat, trying to adjust to your new roles as parents, you will begin to lose some of your energy and all three will be ready for a good sleep. It's hard to be separated after such joyful togetherness.

Hospital Stay

How long you'll remain in the hospital depends on your doctor, your hospital, and you. The minimum hospital stay in our case is two hours after the baby is born. In that time, mother and baby can be checked by obstetrician and pediatrician and if everything is well you may be discharged to your own bed at home for the best sleep ever, with baby safe and secure in your arms or in the bassinet beside your bed.

You may prefer a rest in the hospital with nurses to help you take care of your baby and your meals brought to you on a tray. Rooming-in allows you the opportunity to keep your baby with you constantly while you have an experienced nurse to call if you need help.

The usual hospital stay is about three days. Very often, mother and baby will stay overnight and go home in twenty-four hours. Since hospitals charge by the day, you have paid for one day anyway! You will be guided by the standards in your community and your doctor's wishes, but you make the decision.

I remained in the hospital for three days after Joe's birth. I did not enjoy it at all. The hospital care was great, the food delicious, and the nurses superior, but I did not like being a patient. It was not easy to sleep in a strange bed with light and noise down the hall. I had a roommate whose habits were very different from mine and who invariably wanted to talk when I felt like resting or reading. Just as I planned to rest in the afternoon, visitors would arrive. The baby would be brought to me when he was not hungry and so I had to learn to breastfeed with a sleepy baby. The routine of the hospital did not fit my individual needs. I'd never been in a hospital before as a patient, and as an ex-nurse I began to see "hospital rules" in a new light.

By the time Claryss Nan was born, Dr. Bradley and Dr. Bartlett had established a new rule. If all was well, we could go home after two hours. That was the length of hospital stay that suited me!

If you plan to do the same, I must warn you of a few things. First, it will be assumed by all that you are an exhibitionist who is taking chances with your health and the life of your baby. I was told by an old country doctor that in twenty years I'd see what a foolish thing I had done. I knew he was wrong, but it was such a cruel thing to say to a new mother. Secondly, you may have to post a notice to keep your privacy. You come home early to rest and have your baby where he belongs—in the family. That does not include all the neighbors' children and their pets—at least not for a week or so.

Going Home

Whether you come home in two hours or five days, you should have some help. A grandmother to feed and love the other children and the proud papa, or some paid help to come in for a few hours each morning and tidy up the house. Hire a young girl in the neighborhood to visit after school and play with your toddler for an hour while you and the new baby have a relaxing bath and change clothes to be fresh when Daddy comes home. Soup and a sandwich will be a banquet if you feel rested and charming and the baby is not screaming through dinner. Perhaps your husband doesn't mind bringing home take-out dinners for a few days. You need some time to enjoy and get used to being a new mother before you return to your role of manager of a household. You are not sick, but you *are* a new mother with a babe in her arms. You need care and attention and help for a while. Fathers, pay up—it's a bargain. A contented mother—you know all that!

Review

Now, while you have at least a month until your expected date, you must use your time wisely with practice sessions. Each night before going to sleep you could "pretend labor" for a few minutes. Together, do your relaxing. Make sure that your abdominal breathing is as slow and big and loose as possible. Let your coach check you for one-and-one-half-minute practice sessions. Make sure your position is perfect in every detail. Have your husband run through his relaxation coaching so that he becomes sure of himself and doesn't feel self-conscious with the words that make you feel loose and relaxed. Talk it over, then try again. If you will practice every night from now till labor begins, you will be a good team, ready to handle what your baby has in store for you.

After you've done three or four "relaxing contractions," move on to "pushing" practice. Again, get yourself into position. The easiest way to assume a forty-five-degree squat is with your husband-coach's help. Husbands, kneel on the floor or bed, sitting on your heels. Now your wife can sit at your knees with her back leaning against you. You provide a contour backrest for your wife. Now, practice breath holding. Do not push, since that could contribute to hemorrhoids. Your pushing muscles are strong enough from your lifetime use anyway. The same muscles are used to expel a baby as to expel the contents of the bowel. During practice, then, hold your breath, but *don't push!* Take a first breath—pull your legs apart and toward your shoulders—put chin on chest and hold your breath as long as possible—lift chin—let your breath out fully—take another deep breath, chin on chest, and hold—let your breath out and relax. While you are pushing, your husband is verbally coaching: "Keep chin on chest; hold your breath; push down hard; you're doing fine," etc. A good length of time to practice for a pushing contraction is one and one-half to two minutes. That is quite long and will make the actual labor rather easy.

I've indicated these practice contractions in the order you'll experience them in real labor. But if you're going to get to sleep after practicing, you might be advised to reverse their order and relax after pushing; then you'll be all ready for a good night's sleep. Perhaps your husband deserves a practice session of relaxing and backrub, too, after his work coaching you.

You'll teach each other what is the best relaxing routine by practicing on each other. You must do your bedtime pelvic rocks anyway, so here's a possible routine: Practice pushing together—practice husband-coached relaxing—wife relaxes the coach—wife does pelvic rocking as husband falls asleep—wife gets into bed and falls asleep. You will have to decide who turns out the light and when!

With all this practice, you will be a super team. You'll be ready for your "Olympics" ahead.

You need to be ready for your trip to the hospital. Pack a small suitcase with your essential needs: gown, robe, slippers, toothbrush and toothpaste, and hair-grooming needs. If you like, you can come home in a gown and robe, but if you want to dress, you may want to take a nonmaternity outfit with you—not too tight-fitting, though, as it will take a week or two to get into your usual clothes, maybe longer. For the baby you'll need a warm blanket, rubberized pad (so the wet diaper won't wet you, too), undershirt, nightgown, diapers and pins (or disposable diapers). You probably have a brand new hand-knit outfit from Grandma, so you may use that if you want.

Now you have your bag packed and under your bed, ready for that exciting day when labor begins!

POSTPARTUM

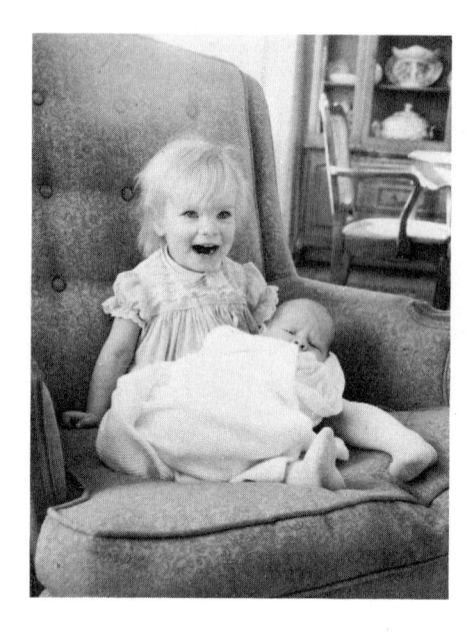

Being Parents
Being a Contented Mother
Tummy Tightener
Waist Trimmer
Being a Wife

Being Parents

Now you are parents! We concentrated so hard on *having* the baby that we neglected your new roles as mother and father. You've had some discussion on what sort of parents you want to be, I'm sure, but have you done anything more than make pronouncements such as "My kid won't . . ." or "I'm certainly not going to allow . . ."? This is serious business. You have a built-in pattern of parenting from your own parents. Do you want to be that same parent? You will probably want to change some aspects! Unfortunately it's a hard pattern to change. Parenting is often more emotional than you intend.

You may want an extra session of the childbirth-training class to discuss being parents. It would be a forum for exploring your values and ideas with others. You will learn from each other. La Leche League will give you involvement with other parents, too (and there is a fathers' meeting). Margie and Jay Hathaway are conducting couples' La Leche meetings in their home in Sherman Oaks, California. You might want to explore that idea in your area.

You will fall into fewer bad habits if you continue to discuss your values as parents together as your child and family grow. I feel that each generation has the responsibility to improve the quality of its children to some degree. You'll do that with good parenting.

There are many good sources of reading which I hope you will pursue. Don't take for granted that you will be the perfect parent that you want to be. You will not! You are a victim of your own emotions. You have bad days and good. Some things will upset you for reasons not even consciously known to you.

There are so many variables. Dick always said to Joe, our oldest, when he became old enough to complain about some fatherly rule, "I'm doing my best, Joe. Remember that I've never been a father before." As a matter of fact, Richard is a fantastic father, and I believe that his success secret is the statement I've quoted. He treats each child with respect and love and each experience on its own merits. He tries to be consistent but is not afraid to be flexible.

Children, even babies, respond very well to honesty. Those may be the standards Dick and I have set as parents—respect and honesty. We hope that our children go into the world able to cope with life and will derive a certain degree of happiness and fulfillment. We feel very strongly the awesome responsibility of our role as parents.

That first day after the baby is born is one of rest for all of you —baby, mother, and father, too. You may be home or you may be in the hospital, as we've discussed. In either place, you will leave the housekeeping details to someone else and concentrate on your baby.

A crying baby is a challenge to you, its mother. Is he wet? Is he hungry? Is he uncomfortable? (Is a pin sticking him? Is a sharp edge of plastic from his disposable diaper cutting into his skin? Is his position wrong?) Try one possible solution after another until your baby is secure again. Perhaps he simply needed your touch. He's been in constant contact with you for nine months; do you wonder that he cries when he wakens alone in a hard, dry, cold bassinet?

Please do not worry about "spoiling" your baby. You can *indulge* an older child, and he may become an unhappy and unpleasant little creature, but you can't *spoil* a child with love. It is perfectly normal and O.K. for a baby to cry. It's not O.K. for you to ignore his cry in the ridiculous attempt to "not spoil" him! Your baby will cry sometimes when you honestly cannot get to him for a few minutes, but he should have the security of knowing that his cry *will* be answered. Can you imagine the hopelessness of a baby whose only means of calling for help is ignored?

When a baby cries he has a need. Fulfill it and the baby will not cry. Respect his need for help; he has no other way to ask. You begin that very first day of your child's life by respecting him as an individual with his own very specific needs.

There may be times when you honestly can't solve the problem. You try every way you know how and the baby cries. You know he's not sick; you've fed, changed, checked, walked, burped, sung to, danced with, and rocked him. You still have a crying baby. (A rare case, it is true.) By now you begin to lose perspective. It's easy to feel that the baby is no longer respecting you! At this point it's up to Daddy to help. "Save me from my child" is a valid need on the part of the mother. Amazingly, the baby may settle down right away with a calm father. If the father is not home, how about a walk outside with baby in his carriage? Go to a neighbor's for coffee—or be honest with her and go for help!

I guess what I want to say to you young mothers is—don't be ashamed of not knowing how. None of us knows how. We learn gradually and there's no right and wrong. Every mother on your block would love to offer help. That's what mothers do best. Be humble enough to ask for help when you really need it. You'll make a friend because she'll be flattered.

Make sure you have at least one person you can call on the phone, to ask her over for coffee or just to visit for a few minutes. Become close enough friends that you could call her at midnight if you needed her.

If you stroll down the street with a baby in a baby carriage, you'll make a friend! It's lovely that human beings of all ages respond to babies as they do.

That first day, after you've rested, you may be overprotective of your baby. He will make "mewing" noises as he moves in his sleep, but don't disturb him. When he really needs you he will cry. It will be a funny noise, but unmistakably a cry. Before many days you'll begin to know the various kinds of cry he makes. It's different for his various needs. A frantic baby will make a frantic cry. And there will be an "I'm beginning to be hungry" cry. You and your child will develop a close communication very quickly. When you have a busy, mixed-up day, do not expect the baby to be quiet and peaceful. Your emotions are too apparent to a breastfed baby.

You will have been to a La Leche League session by now so you know about early breastfeeding and will have a phone number to call if you have any problems. If there is no L.L.L. in your area, be sure you have a copy of *The Womanly Art of Breastfeeding,* the L.L.L. manual for mothers. You'll love reading it as you nurse your baby.

You will work into a routine with your baby and the days will go by very quickly. Do not be surprised if you have some emotional ups and downs. Your body is going through a very big change in these days and you may find yourself crying over burned biscuits or getting mad at your husband because he left the milk out overnight. Again, I plead with that new father and long-suffering husband for just a bit of extra patience. After ten days or two weeks, your wife will be more like herself again.

When the baby is a month or six weeks old, you will need to return to your doctor for a postpartum checkup (find out from him when he wants you to return). He will examine you vaginally to determine your return to normal. Now you may consider yourself ready for any activity you choose!

Being a Contented Mother

To be a good mother and a good wife, you need stimulation of some kind. The mother who has a job will have that. The mother who quits work to be a full-time mother must seek it.

Let us divide your needs into two types, physical and mental.

For your need of physical stimulation, I suggest you join some group where total body exercises will keep your figure in shape and keep you feeling great. The YWCA and YMCA usually have very good fitness programs for a nominal amount of money. If you pay for something, you'll be less likely to skip. Often the adult classes have nursery arrangements, too. Any big community will have privately taught dance classes; modern dance and ballet are marvelous for figure and self-image. Yoga is very popular and you can find classes in it in most communities. You could organize your own program. Invite several friends—or even one—to join you and get a record or a book and "do your own thing." Make it a regular and definite commitment so that you will have a worthwhile exercise program going on. TV offers some exercise programs, too. It's always more fun if you have a friend or a group and can exercise together. Take bike hikes, play tennis, or go swimming. Exercise stimulates your circulation so that you feel invigorated, think better, and have more energy. You can't afford to go without it!

You also need stimulating mentally. You cannot stay at home all day—every day—with a baby who does not talk and expect to be a scintillating conversationalist when your husband comes home from work. Is it any wonder that we grab him and say "Talk to me" when he comes in the door. Usually your husband will ask what has happened throughout your day. You will tell about the cute things that the baby has done—he loves to hear them. Then he'll tell you of the conference he attended or the talk he had with a man who is inventing a new gadget or he might even make the mistake of mentioning the secretary he took to lunch—and you do not love to hear it! His life sounds too exciting and interesting. Your life is so dull. You understand Women's Lib and its fight for the suppressed female. What young full-time mother of one or more small children does not understand the need for Women's Lib at least once in a while?

Now wait a minute! Aren't you doing what you want to do? Of course you are! You have chosen to stay at home and devote these years to your children. Now you must satisfy your need for mental stimulation while you are a mother. You must include in your life activities that are interesting and exciting and that fit in with being a mother. How much better if when you tell your husband about the cute things the baby has done, you can add that you and a neighbor had read the same book and discussed it over the back fence. That you have decided to invite two friends and begin a book-discussion group. Or that you've enrolled in a course on psychology at the local college, or that you and a friend took your babies for a walk in their buggies and picked weeds to make into dried flower arrangements. The possibilities are endless. Whatever you have an urge to do or to study or to learn—now is the time. Your day is yours to plan. Naps and feeding are fairly flexible with babies and young children. You develop a tolerance for "childnoise" and can concentrate despite it. Sometimes you can arrange a baby-sitter or nursery situation to fit your needs. You have no valid excuse for not doing things you want to do.

Find another young mother and do things together. Classes on any craft, art, or handiwork are probably available or at least a book on "how to" could be found for your special interest. Classes in an intellectual pursuit can be taken at almost any college or school (most school districts offer adult education). Your church undoubtedly has discussion groups and learn-how classes. The YMCA and YWCA have a vast variety of programs. If you live in the country or in a very small community, be ingenious and organize a group to do what you would like. You know your own need, so fill it. Don't expect your husband to do it for you. It's not his problem, it's yours. You'll be happier, your husband will be delighted, and your baby will grow up in a secure, comfortable environment.

Or you may be so happy and so content and so fulfilled in your new role as a mother that you do not want to do anything else. That is marvelous. As long as you are satisfied with your life, don't try to change it.

I channeled my energies into childbirth teaching as soon as Joe was born and it's been a perfect solution. I taught one or two evenings a week, when Richard could baby-sit and the children were in bed. As well as teaching these classes, I became a leader of L.L.L. These were evening meetings in my own home and usually only once a month. There's no better way of meeting people, of having mental stimulation, and of helping others. Along with that I began going to a once-a-week class in modern dancing, belonged to a discussion group, took mandolin lessons and swimming lessons. Very quickly I had expanded to the point where I was *too* stimulated and needed to spend more time at home keeping things in order. I am a firm believer in arranging my time so that my family comes first. When I forget, Dick and the children remind me!

If you are devoting ten to twenty years of your life to being a mother, you must also be a fulfilled individual. Do what is necessary to maintain your own self-image.

Lynn Rimel, one of our Denver teachers, is an expert on what facilities of interest the community offers. She became involved in many activities, some with her daughter, Wendy, and some without. Finally Lynn decided that she needed the stimulation of working again. So she took a part-time secretarial job, three days a week. It was a successful experiment for Lynn because she realized that she'd much rather be at home with Wendy and has now gone back to full-time mothering (to the extent of being pregnant). You may need to find out, as Lynn did, if you really want to be a working mother. Some of you may indeed want to be.

Let me warn you against waiting until your children are in school to do all those many things you want to do. Our five children are all

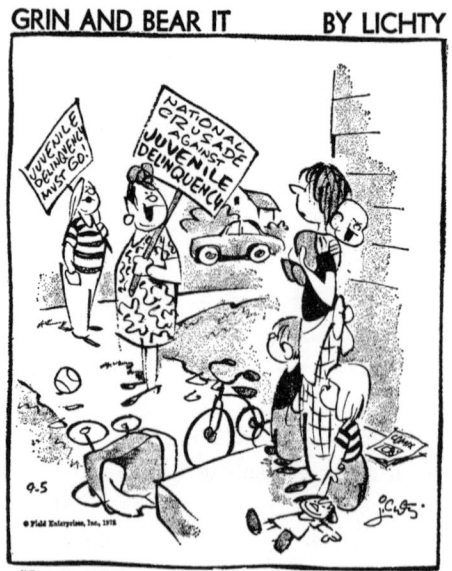

"Surely, Adele, you can find a place to dump the kids somewhere and give us a hand with such a worthy cause!"

in school now and I have no more spare time than I ever had. It's different mothering, but not less busy.

You will have to take care of your own "mental stimulation" programs. All I can do is encourage you. But I do have some definite help for you as to your physical activity—Mabel Lumm Fitzhugh's postpartum exercises, which I learned from her. They are marvelous. They're specific for that part of you which was stretched out of shape while you were pregnant, and they do not require too much energy; so they are perfect for the first six weeks postpartum (after delivery of the baby). During this six weeks, you should also be doing at least eighty pelvic rocks a day to get the uterus into the correct position in your body—involution of the uterus—as you firm and tighten up.

You may have a vaginal discharge for up to six weeks. It's bloody for the first ten days or so and then becomes a dark brown. It is drainage from the healing uterus and is very normal.

I often forget to mention "after-birth pains," which are just what it says. They are a minimal problem with natural childbirth deliveries. For up to five days after the birth, you will feel the uterus as it contracts back down to its normal size. The contractions may be very strong and quite unpleasant. Your doctor will probably give you a stronger-than-aspirin type of drug to take if you need to. By coincidence, I discovered that the postpartum exercises seemed to relieve the worst afterbirth pains that I had. However, even with our fifth, Ritchie, my uterus contracted with so little pain that I did not take even an aspirin. Never did I fill the prescription that the doctor gave me. It is generally expected that after-birth pains are worse with each baby. If you are uncomfortable, use the drug that was given you. But try the postpartum exercises first!

We have given you some postures and exercises for pregnancy which we hope you will incorporate into your daily life forever!

Pelvic rocks should be done every day. About forty to eighty will do. Before bed is still the best time, and on hands and knees. It will keep your uterus in the proper place, your abdominal muscles firm, and your back strong.

Standing pelvic rock has taught you to maintain that perfect posture. Use it always.

Tailor sitting is still the best possible sitting position—pregnant or not.

Squatting makes sense when you must get to the floor to reach anything. Now that you are not pregnant, you may want to use your legs to come up and not tip your body forward. It's up to you.

Kegels must be maintained throughout life for all the reasons given previously—twenty per hour while you are awake.

Hopefully, you will use the relaxation techniques to make your life more calm. It helps when you are under stress. Here now are the postpartum exercises I've been promising.

Tummy Tightener—
Postpartum Exercise One

This will tighten all the parts of you stretched from your pregnancy. Your abdomen, thighs, Kegel, and bottom—the area of your body that needs to be returned to normal—will be tensed as you do this exercise. The rest of your body should have remained in good condition throughout your pregnancy, if you were maintaining reasonable exercise.

This is a good tummy tightener for all women who have lost the muscle tone in their abdomen.

HOW To start, lie flat on your back. Cross your legs at the knees and put your hands on your abdomen. Now tighten in four ways:

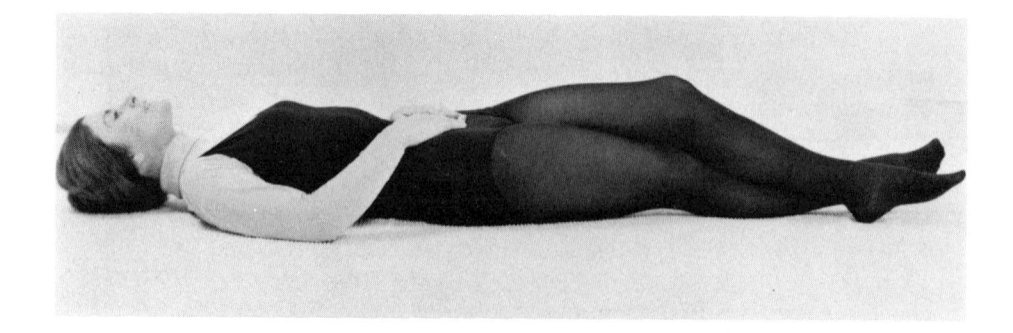

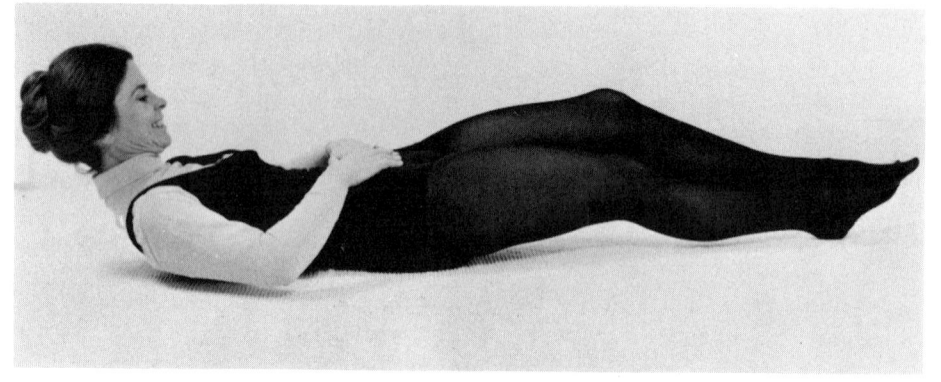

1. Roll both knees toward each other, tightening the inner thigh. Hold.
2. Do a Kegel. Hold.
3. Raise your head until you feel your abdominal muscles tighten under your fingers. Hold.
4. Squeeze your buttocks. Hold.
5. Release everything and relax.

Now repeat. Each of you will have your own "required" number of times. Some women have done it one hundred times a day and *really* look great. If twenty a day keeps you firm, then that is fine. Perhaps it will take more or less, but find your own maintenance requirement.

WHERE All you need is a flat surface. You may even lie on your bed, though a carpeted floor is better.

WHEN Have eight hours' sleep after the baby is born and then begin a few postpartum exercises. Work very slowly so as not to make yourself stiff and sore. Space these exercises throughout the day at comfortable intervals. I suggest that you work up to fifty a day by six weeks after the baby is born. If you want to do more, that is fine.

When I have been lazy and my abdominal muscles get loose and flabby, I do thirty to fifty of these—plus the next postpartum exercise, which goes with it—and in two days I can tell the difference. It really works and fast!

The beauty of these exercises is that they can both be done as you go to bed at night because they are easy and quiet and you'll be able to fall asleep afterward (when can't a new mother fall asleep?). They do not necessarily invigorate you, as so many exercises do. I usually forget to exercise until I am in bed at night, so these are a blessing to me.

Waist Trimmer— Postpartum Exercise Two

This exercise, specifically for the waist and midriff as well as the abdomen, is the completion of the first postpartum exercise. The two should always be done together.

This will help you button your waistbands again!

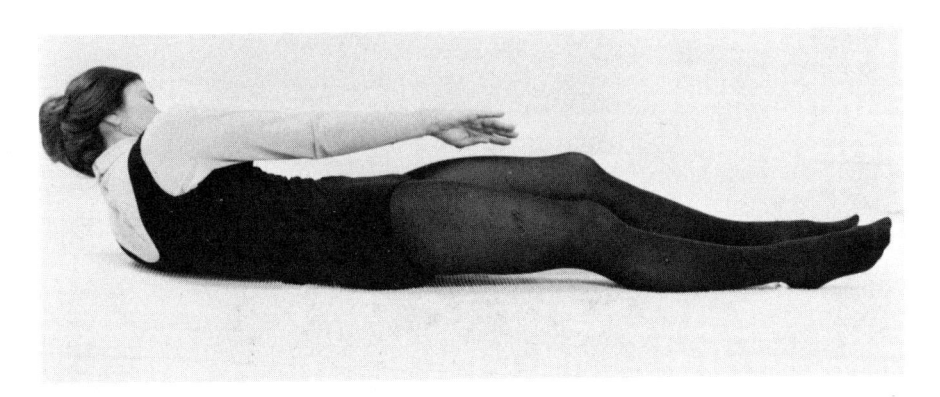

HOW

1. Lie flat on your back on a padded floor. Bend one knee slightly —about four inches from the bottom of your knee to the floor.
2. With the opposite hand, point toward the raised knee. Your head is raised and your one shoulder. You can feel the pull through your waist.
3. Relax.
4. Bend the other knee slightly and point toward it with the opposite hand and shoulder.

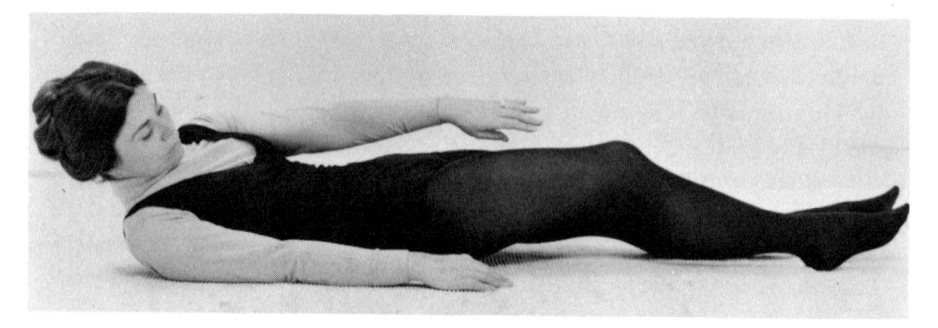

5. Relax.
6. Do your "required" number of times—equal number to postpartum exercise one.

If you can touch your knee with your hand, you are a contortionist, or your arms are very long, or you have your knee raised too high!

WHERE On the same surface as postpartum exercise one.

WHEN At the same time as postpartum exercise one.

Being a Wife

Remember, you are a wife as well as a mother!

Now that you are a family, you must keep the unit strong. To do that you must never lose sight of what brought the two of you together in the first place. As you mature and change and grow and develop as individuals, so should your love for each other. When my children ask, "Who do you love best, Mommy?" (as all of them have), I always say, "I love you five equally and I love Daddy best. I was given you, but I picked Daddy." The children don't like the answer but Daddy does! It's important for children to grow up in an environment where love is apparent. I'm not talking about a sterile and gooey and sweet situation. Two individuals must have some disagreements, but arguing is very different from hating! Even being angry is not hating.

I have found that the day goes much more smoothly if you organize around "coming-home time for Daddy." A nap is a must for mother and baby (or babies). Mother does not need to sleep but could lock her door for an hour to sew or read or create or do nothing. You need to be alone. When you've had your hour, it's easier to make Dad's first hour home pleasant. Greet him! You're glad to see him, so show it.

I know, he always gets there just as you meant to finish tidying up or before you put on lipstick. Try to be ready early, but if you aren't, a warm greeting will help overcome the effect of a messy, toy-strewn living room. The hour before dinner should be for Dad. If he likes to play with the children, then it would be perfect, but usually he'd rather visit quietly with you, read the paper, or watch the news. Respect his need and help create a home in which he can relax.

Hungry children are unpleasant, so let them have a healthful snack in the late afternoon to tide them over to dinner. It can be considered the first course. You and your husband, too, may want to relax with a drink or snack. You could serve the children soup at 5 P.M. and have dinner at 6 P.M. Children's TV programs are usually timed to create a buffer time zone for parents. A brand-new baby is no problem, as you and your husband can visit or watch the news together while the baby breastfeeds. Don't be surprised if this is baby's "fussy time" (there has to be one span of time when even a newborn baby stays awake). It's only a fussy time if the baby is bored. It's the time for talking, singing, and playing with your baby. That's how he'll learn, by your playing with and talking to him. So with proper stimulation, "fussy time" is "happy time." Daddy can join in and share this delightful period.

As the children get older, the playing changes. It gets more and more active and father and child build up a communication through these fun-filled times together. Fathers will look forward to that time in their day as much as the children. Swinging and tickling turns into hide-and-seek. Tag is the big father-child sport in our house now, and it can get very wild. I never play—that's Dad's game! The older the children get, the less physical the games become. We are gradually getting into conversations with the older ones, rather than games.

Back to taking care of Daddy when he gets home from work. Obviously, if you treat him right every evening when he's exhausted, he's going to reward you, right? Right! Maybe he'll make a dinner date with you for one evening each week and relieve you of the wifely duties at home. You'll get a baby-sitter and dress up in his favorite dress and go out on the town. Sometimes you'll go to a movie or out with friends, but don't forget to have some quiet "alone" evenings when you can talk. As I've mentioned, the hardest thing for parents is to talk to each other. There's always a little one listening in!

You know how to tell married from nonmarried couples at a restaurant, don't you? The married couples don't talk. It's up to us married couples to prove that dumb joke wrong! So keep your friendship strong and active. To do that you need to be together alone sometimes. As a matter of fact, you need to take the whole thing one step further. You need to be alone overnight once in a while. We have been fortunate in always taking at least a weekend trip alone during each year. How we enjoy it! And how we need it! Try to spend a day or two away from your children occasionally. It's important for all of you. The children will benefit and so will you parents. You may not have a baby-sitter who can take over at your house, so try a trade-off with friends. It's awful when you double the family for a weekend—but it's worth it when your turn comes and you leave your children with the other family. You may simply stay at home, have a candlelight dinner with no little voices interrupting, or you may have saved for a swank resort weekend. Whatever you do, it will make you appreciate each other and will give you the perspective to realize the excitement and fun of your role as parents. The children will learn to be more flexible and will begin to trust Mommy and Daddy to leave *and* return again. It's their vacation, too, if they stay with grandparents or their own buddies. You are all building toward the future when the child will leave home to "make his way in the world" and the parents are alone again, the way it all began.

A Letter to My Sister

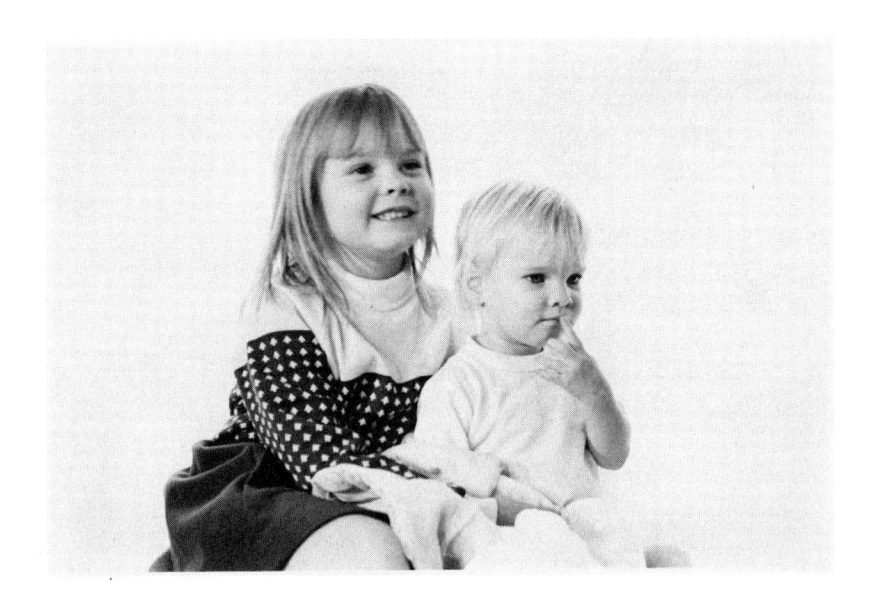

This is an actual letter written to my only sister, Clarice Siebens, and her husband, Bill, in Calgary, Alberta, when they were expecting their first child, Carter. They now have two more, Rhondda and Evann. The doctor was helpful and the birth experiences were happy. I include it because it was the actual beginning of this book.

Dear Clarice & Bill:

How I wish you could be here to have your baby with us where we have classes, sympathetic doctors, and a hospital that allows couples to stay together for a birth. Naturally you are concerned. Childbirth is such an "unknown" with your first baby. Read the books I've recommended. Remember the talks we've had about my childbirth experiences. Now, here are some last-minute reminders to help you be ready for the most exciting thing that will ever happen to you both.

For *pregnancy* and back comfort, the pelvic rock is best. Standing posture is extremely important—hold your pelvis level rather than letting the baby's weight pull your tummy out and your back into a sway. Do eighty pelvic rocks on all fours just before bed *every* night. No matter how tired you are, do those bedtime pelvic rocks! It is easy enough to work in the other pelvic rocks when it's convenient during the day.

Get off your feet and put them up as often as possible even though you may not feel the need. Varicose veins run in our family, and it's almost a normal thing with pregnancy.

For labor, become proficient at abdominal breathing and relaxing. These *may* take a great deal of control and effort as your labor progresses, so practice as soon as you feel contractions—even though not hard ones—so you'll be an old hand at it by late first stage. This is all you do throughout your whole first-stage labor—relax and tummy-breathe with each contraction. Be sure to breathe *out* as completely as *in* to prevent hyperventilation, which makes your fingers get stiff during labor and is easily cured by breathing into a paper bag, or cupped hands, so you breathe some carbon dioxide.

We find that the time for the most control on your part is transition, or when the cervix is seven to ten centimeters dilated. Carry on with abdominal breathing and *complete* relaxation. Here it helps if you have something to think about, for example, the picture Nita Wolf painted for me of the clouds and view from Jungfrau Joch—these are what I used—as well as Richard's reassurance and encouragement: "You are doing fine, things are going well, let yourself relax," etc. This transition is a relatively short time in labor—trickiest but shortest!

Second stage is pushing and you have no choice in the matter. Your body lets you do *nothing* else, so don't resist but work with it. It's automatic and it's marvelous. This is where you will be *expected* to "take something" and this is where the fun comes in. You work hard but if you will raise your head, as though trying to see the baby coming, and push hard enough, you will have no pain—honest. This does not require any "control," only hard pushing such as you'd do with a very constipated bowel movement, only harder work. (I hate to say that except it's one way for you to know *how* to push!) Take a deep breath and hold it while you push. Let it out in a gush when you can't hold your breath any longer, take another big chest breath, and keep pushing as long as there is any contraction. The doctor may have to tell you when to stop pushing, as sometimes it's not definite to you but he can see when the contraction is over.

Plead with your doctor to read Dr. Bradley's book so that his help can be more than to "offer you something." What you'll need is encouragement, *not* gas, so that you can be awake to push and for the excitement of the birth!

In case your doctor asks you: yes, we do episiotomies, and the pressure of crowning and pushing makes its own natural anesthetic for the cutting (midline usually, if possible), but a local is given for suturing after the birth of the baby.

Richard's word for Bill: do not worry if labor is long. It can go on for hours and hours and be very normal. Apparently he became worried with Joey, as it took fifteen hours all told—but I was too busy relaxing and enjoying a new experience to realize he was worried, and he, bless him, did not tell me! The advantage of a long labor is that you get good at everything as you go along! *Expect* it to be long, then you'll not be disappointed. (Fifteen hours is not long, but it is with natural childbirth.)

Gosh, I wish I could talk with you. I'm not trying to *tell* you what to do unless this is what you want in the first place. Anything that makes your experiences in childbirth happy and pleasant cannot be failure, no matter how far you go with our methods. I am convinced that a happy labor changes your general attitude to the children and your husband.

Another point—when you are pushing, you look as though you are in pain. The picture of me pushing makes everyone feel sympathy, and maybe this is why they shove gas at you. Of course, it hurts if you *don't* push!

Never, never, never lie flat on your back during labor. They may do your "prep" and leave you lying that way. Either roll over on your side with leg drawn up and arm behind you or in a contour, half-sitting/half-lying position on your back (hospital beds crank into this position at knee and back), with pillows under your arms or wherever needed to help you be comfy. Change position when you get stiff or uncomfortable. Move about in between contractions, especially until transition.

Rienne cut her "right front top center" tooth today and is a bit fussy. She's so funny—all teeth (seven)—much like Joey as a baby with more hair—not long hair, but really thick.

The other two are sweet as ever. Joey has come out of his "frightful four" stage and is a darling again. Claryss Nan is amazing—we were withholding dessert because she had not eaten her main course, so she rushed off and brought Richard's slippers and put them on. Naturally, she got dessert! She seems to understand the power of a smile, and really throws on the charm!

One more word on natural childbirth before I mail this. It's good for Uncle Bill to know that having a baby requires, more or less, the same amount of energy needed to play four quarters of football—hence the necessity of preparing by exercising in advance. Also, this amount of work, with no half-time break, requires lots of encouragement and help from the coach—namely Bill. He'll be able to stay with you till nearly pushing time probably—and it will be a marvelous help. It's ghastly to be left alone during labor and nurses are usually too busy—and it's dull for them! The only one you'll really want is Bill anyway. At first you can play cards or visit, but later you'll just need to know he's there. Bill —I'm writing this for you. Never will you be more proud of and proud to be with Clarice—so be a good papa. Hold her hand but be firm about her relaxing and tummy breathing. It could be a long time.

Remember, you would be perfect at this if you had perfect circumstances. Any amount of comfort and enjoyment you gain from all this is worth it and if you do things differently from us, that's O.K. It's a glorious experience and it's the end result that's best of all! (Writing this all down makes me ready to have another.)

Love and kisses,
Your big sis,
Rhondda

INDEX

Abdominal breathing, 134; during pregnancy, 39; in labor, 39; and relaxation, 33, 36–39
Abdominal muscles, exercises to tighten, 25–29, 127–130
Abductor muscles, exercises to strengthen, 61–63
After-birth pains, 85
American Academy of Husband-Coached Childbirth, 16
Amniotic sac, breaking of, in labor, 98–99
Ankles, flexing and stretching, 75–77

Baby, newborn, 121–123
Back, exercises to strengthen, 55–61, 134
Baghdady, Anna and Hesham, 109–110
Bartlett, Dr. Max D., 3, 8–9, 117
Bergren, Stephanie, 9, 10
Blood circulation. See Circulation
"Bloody show," 99–100
Bradley, Dr. Robert A., 2–3, 8–9, 29, 30, 39, 46, 79, 85, 109, 117
Braxton Hicks contractions, 100
Brewer, Dr. Thomas, 48
Breastfeeding, 82–88; advantages of, 83–86; allergies and, 87–88; first, 114–115; immediate postpartum, 85–86; immediate postpartum, and after-birth pains, 85; La Leche League and, 82–83, 88, 121–122, 123; milk "coming in" in, 86; nipple care in, 92–94
Breasts: exercises to aid, 88–92; proper support of, 93
Breath holding, for pushing in labor, 77–80
Breathing. See Abdominal breathing
Buchan, Edwina, 1
Bust booster, 88–92; after the birth, 91–92; during pregnancy, 91
Butterfly, 61–63

Cervix. See Labor
Chest posture, exercise to aid, 88–92
Childbirth: emergency, 98. See also Natural childbirth
Circulation: exercises to aid, 25–29, 40–44, 55–61. See also Varicose veins
Contractions: in beginning labor, 96–97; beginning of, 97–98; Braxton Hicks, 100; "practice," 118

Danneberg, Florence, 12
Davis, Adelle, 48–49
Delivery. See Labor
Deutsch, Ronald M., 66
Dick-Read, Grantly, 1
Diet in pregnancy, 48–52

Emergency Childbirth, 98
Episiotomy: exercise to aid healing of, 65–68; repair of, 115. See also Labor, second-stage

False labor, 100–101
Fitzhugh, Mabel Lumm, 9, 58–59; postpartum exercises of, 127–130
Foot circles, 73–75
Freese, Kathy, 83
French, Mrs. Arlene, 84

Hartman, Allison Lucille, 14, 88; birth of, 11–13
Hartman, Claryss Nan, 10, 14, 117, 135–136; birth of, 9
Hartman, Grandmother, 9, 13
Hartman, Joseph Baden (Joe), 10, 11, 14, 87, 116, 121, 125, 135; birth of, 2–9
Hartman, Richard, 2, 3, 4, 5, 6–8, 10, 12, 13–14, 30, 87, 97, 121, 125, 134, 135
Hartman, Richard Evans (Ritchie), 87; birth of, 13–14
Hartman, Rienne Frances, 9, 14; birth of, 10–11
Hathaway, Margie and Jay, 121

Heartburn, 47–48; exercises to relieve, 88–92
Hemorrhoids, exercise to prevent, 65–68
Hospital: going home from, 117; stay, after delivery, 116–117; stay, preparation for, 119
Husband-Coached Childbirth, 39, 46

Kegel, Dr. Arnold, 65–66, 67
Kegel exercise, 65–68, 127
Kegel muscle, 78; exercises to tighten, 65–68, 127–129
Kerwin, Mary Ann, 9, 10, 12, 30
Kerwin, Tom, 9, 30
Key to Feminine Response in Marriage, The, 66
Knees, flexing and stretching, 75–77

Labor: abdominal breathing and relaxation in, 134; contractions in, 96–97; delivery, 113–114; delivery, contracting of uterus after, 115; dilation of cervix in, 102, 109, 134; effacement of cervix in, 102; false, 100–101; first-stage, 101–104; practice for, 103–104; review of, 117–119, 134–135; second-stage, 109–113; second-stage, episiotomy in, 112–113, 135; second-stage, in multipara, 111; second-stage, in primipara, 110–111; second-stage, pushing in, 109–113; signs of, 97–101; third-stage, 115; transition in, 104–106, 134
La Leche League. *See* Breastfeeding
Landers, Ann, 84
Leg cramps, 46–47
Leg elevation, 70–73
Legs, exercises to stretch, 21–25, 75–77
Leg stretches, 75–77
List, Debbie, 61
List, Kelly, 61

McCutcheon, Gary and Sue, 112
Mijer, Dr., 9, 12, 13
Monilia, prevention of, 21, 41
Motherhood, coping with, 121–127
Mulloy, Mary (Mrs. James Hawk), 2

Natural childbirth: definition of, 18–19; importance of abdominal breathing in, 37–38; importance of exercises in, 20–21; importance of relaxation in, 30; role of doctor in, 19, 20; role of husband in, 19; role of wife in, 19
Nausea, 16
Nipple care, 92–94
Nursing. *See* Breastfeeding
Nursing Your Baby, 85

Obstetrics ward, visit to, 101–102

Parenthood, 121–123
Pelvic rock, 24–29; kitchen sink, 58–61; as postpartum exercise, 126–127; rest position during, 29; sitting, 53–55; standing, 55–58, 127; variations, 53–60
Pelvis, pressure on, exercises to relieve, 53–55, 58–61
Perineum, exercise to stretch, 40–44
Placenta, expulsion of, 115
Postpartum period, 121–132; physical characteristics of, 126–127
Posture, exercises to aid, 25–29, 55–58, 88–92; in lifting, 43–44.
Pregnancy: advice and "old wives' tales" in, 17, 19–20; and choosing a doctor, 16–17; diet in, 48–52; general characteristics of, 15–18, 45–46, 64–65, 81–82, 95–96, 107–108; leg cramps in, 46–47; nausea in, 16; relationship of husband and wife in, 17; sex life in, 17, 108; varicose veins in, 68–70
Pryor, Karen, 85
Pubococcygeus muscle. *See* Kegel muscle
Pushing: breathing for, 77–80; practice, avoiding, 80

Ratner, Dr. H., 17
Recovery room, 115–116
Relaxation, 29–36, 134; and abdominal breathing, 33, 36–39; classic position in, 31; classic position in, variation, 32; contour position in, 32; poem for, 34–35; proper conditions for, 33
Rice, Peggy, 4, 9, 28
Rimel, Lynn, 84, 125
Rimel, Wendy, 125

Scutt, Linda, 75
Sex life, in pregnancy, 17, 108
Siebens, Bill, 133–138
Siebens, Carter, 133
Siebens, Clarice, 133–138

Siebens, Evann, 133
Siebens, Rhondda, 133
Squat, 40–44, 127; getting up from, 41; lifting posture in, 43–44

Tailor sit, 21–25, 127; variations, 22–23
Tennes, Katherine, 13
Tension, exercises to relieve, 25–36, 53–55
Thighs, exercise to tighten, 127–129
Transition. *See* Labor
Tummy tightener, 127–129

Uterus: contracting of, after delivery, 115; prolapse of, exercise to prevent, 65–68; prolapse of, symptoms of, 66–67

Varicose veins, 68–70; exercises to prevent, 25–29, 55–61, 69–77. *See also* circulation

Waist trimmer, 129–130
White, Dr. Gregory, 98
Wife, being a, in motherhood, 130–132
Wolf, Nita, 134
Womanly Art of Breastfeeding, The, 82–83, 88, 123